A tragic but inspiring journey through life. Strength and faith are spelled "**Dravecky**."

> Al Rosen, President and General Manager
> San Francisco Giants

Dave Dravecky is an inspiration to me, as he has been to everyone whose life he has touched. *When You Can't Come Back* is an outstanding sequel to *Comeback*. This latest book is the story of how a man and his family have dealt with and are dealing with situations most people would have a hard time handling.

> Roger Craig, Manager
> San Francisco Giants

If you've ever experienced pain and cried out, "Why me?" Dave and Jan Dravecky have been there. They were forced to trade a baseball career full of promise, for a season of life filled with pain. In *When You Can't Come Back*, you won't find worn-out cliches, or "surefire steps" to breeze through life's difficulties. But you will find an inspiring story, deeply felt insights, and an unshakable faith—all put within our reach—that are a breath of fresh air. We highly recommend this book.

> Gary Smalley and John Trent
> *Today's Family*

Too many Christians still think that handling tough times requires little more than read the Bible, trust God, and do what He says. With unusual courage and candor, the Draveckys make clear that *real* victory does not come without terrific struggle, but it does come. Honest people facing life as it is, and finding more of Christ—this is their story.

> Larry and Rachael Crabb

When You Can't Come Back is much more than a sports bio. This book can touch the world with its story of two public people who discovered a simple but profound truth: When our loss is deepest, God is closest. The Draveckys and Ken Gire will help any reader who has ever experienced struggle, failure, or disappointment.

> John Townsend, Ph.D., Clinical Director
> Minirth-Meier Clinic West

Here is a powerful account of how pain and loss can be a door to new life. Dave and Jan give hope to all those who feel they have reached the end.

Henry Cloud, Ph.D.

Dave and Jan replace the "happily-ever-after" myth with a window into their own desperate struggle for survival against staggering opposition. Their story is a gift of hope to the Christian community.

Bill Hybels, Senior Pastor
Willow Creek Community Church

Sports at its best can be a wonderful example of how to live life graciously with its wins and losses. Thank God for models such as Dave Dravecky who, as Kipling says, "meets with Triumph and Disaster and treats those two imposters just the same." *When You Can't Come Back* is a wonderful insight into Dave's triumphal living.

Bill Gaither

Dave Dravecky's first book showed he is a man of courage and faith. His new book shows that he courageously holds to his faith, in spite of trouble and hardship. My hat is off to him.

Tom Landry
Former Head Coach, Dallas Cowboys

Jan and Dave Dravecky's book is a wonderful sharing of trials, tribulations, and an injection of positive courage for the reader.

Peter Ueberroth
Former Commissioner of Baseball

Nothing could better sum up what Dave and Jan are trying to share with us in this book than Philippians 3:14: "I press on toward the goal ..." I encourage you to read the book.

Billy Graham

When You Can't
COME BACK

A Story of Courage & Grace

When You Can't
COME BACK

Dave & Jan Dravecky
with Ken Gire

ZondervanPublishingHouse
Grand Rapids, Michigan

HarperSanFrancisco
San Francisco, California

Divisions of HarperCollinsPublishers

WHEN YOU CAN'T COME BACK
Copyright © 1992 by Dave and Jan Dravecky

Co-published by Zondervan Publishing House
Grand Rapids, Michigan 49530, and HarperSanFrancisco

Library of Congress Cataloging-in-Publication Data

Dravecky, Dave.
    When you can't come back / by Dave and Jan Dravecky, with Ken
Gire.
        p. cm.
    ISBN 0-310-58560-0
    1. Dravecky, Dave—Health. 2. Cancer—Patients—United States–
Biography. 3. Baseball players—United States—Biography.
I. Dravecky, Jan. II. Gire, Ken. III. Title.
RC265.6.D73A3 1992
796.357'092–dc20
    [B]   92–53526
                                                              CIP

Edited by John D. Sloan
Cover designed by Mark Veldheer
Cover photo by Bill Bilsley

Published in association with Sealy M. Yates, Orange, California.

Printed in the United States of America

92 93 94 95 96 / DH / 5   4   3

This edition is printed on acid-free paper and meets the American National Standards Institute Z39.48 standard.

Contents

Acknowledgments

As WE HAVE stepped back and reflected on this manuscript, we have been amazed at how God has been working in our lives for the past three years. Remembering how at times we felt so alone, unable to sense God's presence, we were moved to tears as we could now see that he was always there working through some very special people he had brought into our lives.

Two of those special people are Ken and Judy Gire. Our friendship started way before this book was ever conceived. They were two concerned friends who could see we were struggling and cared enough to help with their time and their counsel. Fortunately, after the amputation, Ken agreed to help us write this book. We are so grateful for the way God has used Ken to tell our story and to contribute to our ministry.

There have been some very special people who made this book possible. Without their support and encouragement we doubt very much if this book would have come to fruition! We would like to thank Scott Bolinder and John Sloan, who are more than just our publisher and editor. They have become good friends, and we are grateful for their counsel and encouragement over these past three years.

We would like to thank George Craig at HarperCollins

and Jim Buick at Zondervan for believing in our story and making it possible to be published.

Where would we be without Sealy and Susan Yates? They have been there through it all, from organizing our busy schedule to making sure that this story got published. More important than all of that, though, has been their love and support for us in the most difficult of times. Thank you so much for being so faithful!

Dr. Brennan and his staff at Memorial Sloan-Kettering Cancer Center have been incredible. With all the respect and admiration we can muster, Thank you!

Dennis Graham and the 16th floor nursing and medical staff made our visits to Memorial Sloan-Kettering most memorable and even wonderful, even in the most difficult of times. Thank you so much for your love and care for us. You made all the difference!

Dr. Charles McGowen was not only our dedicated and caring physician, but he also became our friend, providing very timely and godly counsel.

Our professional help did not stop there. We are so thankful to our friend Dr. John Townsend, co-director of Minirth-Meier Clinic West, who took time for us on that Sunday afternoon in May and turned our lives in the direction for healing. We also are very grateful for Dr. Lorin Sommers. We are eternally thankful to these two men of God for their godly wisdom and love.

When we were in baseball, God always provided special friendships. One of those friendships was Atlee and Jenny Hammaker. No matter the time or space between us, we knew they would always be there and that they will always care. We've called on them a lot over the past three years, and they have indeed been there for us. We love them and are grateful for their faithfulness.

When we moved back to Ohio, retiring from baseball, we were not close to very many people in our hometown, but we knew God would provide new friendships. Once again, he brought many special relationships into our lives. One of them was with Bob and Patty Struharik. They have been through all our trials over the past two years and shared our tears, many times carrying and praying us through the valleys. We thank God for true friendships like theirs. We truly love them both.

We were persuaded by family and friends to establish The Dave Dravecky Foundation as an organization through which we could carry out our ministry of responding to the hurts of so many who have and will call upon us for help. A special thanks to those who have helped include: Bob and Shirley Eddy, Bruce and Phyllis Beard, Dr. Charles and Kay McGowen, Bobby and Patty Struharik, and Sealy and Susan Yates.

We would not want to neglect to say thank you to our families for their love and support through all our struggles: Our children Tiffany and Jonathan, God's incredible gift to us; and my brothers and their wives, Rick and Kathy, Frank and Missy, Joe and Gina. Last, but not least, my baby brother George, who offered to be my official shoe-tier when my arm was amputated.

Writing this book has not been the easiest of things to do. Jan and I have bared our hearts to those of you who would choose to read this story. In the midst of our own pain and suffering we hope that through the pages of this book you would come away feeling encouraged, maybe even set free, but most of all, with a sense of hope, not temporal, but eternal, as you face the days ahead!

Surgical loss of an arm is a tragedy for the patient and failure for the surgeon. The removal of Dave Dravecky's arm was more than the loss of a limb; it was the loss of a part of a life, part of a lifestyle, and part of a particular person's essential being. It is hard to conceive that anything good could come from such a mutilating procedure. As Dave Dravecky tells it, it was another one of the events that has focused his life and the life of his family on what they had to give to the world, rather than on what had been taken away.

For me, it was more complex. That something positive could come from an amputation seemed the antithesis of everything I believed in and was trained to do. Yet somehow, through an inner reserve, Dave has taken the loss of what was up until that time his most important asset, turned it in and then turned it out, and allowed growth, such that the loss has somehow made him greater. Dave Dravecky has shown that adversity can strengthen a relationship, redirect a life, and provide hope and inspiration for all. It has been a privilege for me to have helped in a very tiny piece of this story.

Murray F. Brennan, M.D.
Memorial Sloan-Kettering Cancer Center

Introduction

WHEN I RETIRED from baseball, I thought I had learned all the lessons about life I needed to learn. I looked forward to being off the road and at home with my family, settled down to some kind of normal, 9-to-5 life.

But the past two years have been anything but normal, and I've found out there's still a lot left to learn.

This book is not about a hero. It is about someone very, very human. Two someones, actually, as it is as much Jan's story as it is mine. We take turns in the book as we tell our story.

Our story is less of a book, actually, and more of a journal kept by two weary people who trudged, often out of step with each other, through a desolate wilderness. The past two years were a disorienting time for Jan and me. We went through more surgeries, we struggled with depression, and we finally had to face the amputation of my arm. There was little shade in the wilderness we found ourselves in, and most of the wells along the way were dry.

During that time I was faced with some pretty searing questions. Questions like: What do you do when a part of your life is taken away from you forever? How do you adjust? How do you handle problems of self-esteem and depression? What do you do when no matter how hard you try, how much faith you have, how fervently you pray, things will never return to the way they were? What do you do when you can't change the circumstances of your life?

What do you do when you can't come back?

Sooner or later that's a question we all have to face. For me it just happened to be sooner.

But before I open that chapter of my life, let me take you back thirty years ago to a small town in Ohio where the story first began.

– 1 –

Beginning of the Dream

IT BEGAN IN THE backyard with a game of catch. A game of catch with my dad. He was a machinist and about as blue collar as you could get. Boy, did he ever come home dirty at the end of a day. I still remember him walking through our front door just before dinner and how dark his trousers used to look, smeared with the day's work . . . how he smelled of sweat and grease . . . how the black grime had collected under the fingernails of his hands.

Such big hands, I used to think back then, *such big, strong hands*.

I thought those hands could do anything. And usually they could. If it was broken, he could fix it. I remember how hard those hands worked around the house. I remember a scene of him on a ladder, leaning to paint the eaves of our house. One of him in the kitchen, taking a brush and smoothing out the bubbles of freshly hung wallpaper. Another one of him under the hood of the car, fixing the engine. A scene of him getting the heater ready for winter. Another one of him sprawled out on the bathroom floor, fixing the pipes to the sink.

He could do whatever needed doing around our little house in Boardman, Ohio. As a kid growing up, I felt safe and secure knowing that those big, strong, fix-anything hands belonged to the man I called "Dad."

Regardless how tired those hands got at the end of the day, they were never too tired for a game of catch. In the backyard he'd burrow one of those big, strong hands into a catcher's mitt and play with a seven-year-old boy who could barely wrap his hand around a baseball. I remember how he would crouch down and pound his fist into that mitt, making a well-rounded pocket for the ball I was about to pitch. Often we played till it was too dark to see, and still I begged for more, never wanting that time to end.

It didn't take me long to convert the backyard into a ball diamond where all the neighborhood kids came to play. We wore a beaten path around the trees we used for bases, hit fouls that ricocheted off the house, and knocked homers past the fenceless yards of our neighbors.

The backyard was never the same after my dad first put on that glove and played catch with me.

Neither was I.

I fell in love with the game of baseball. After church our family would stretch out in the living room and watch inning after inning of it on TV. We huddled around our black-and-white set where we cheered the Indians, booed the umpire, and tipped off the infield whenever a batter looked like he was going to bunt. Sometimes Dad's brother Andy would stop by and watch with us. He was a minor league player for the Pittsburgh Pirates. He loved the game, too. I guess it was in the Dravecky blood to love baseball.

Or maybe it was in that backyard. For it was there I first dreamed of being a big-league pitcher.

It wasn't long until I outgrew the backyard to play in

bigger ballfields in Little League, Pony League, and Colt League. During those days I imagined I was Sandy Koufax, flame thrower for the Los Angeles Dodgers. Koufax was my idol. I would sit glued to the TV, memorizing his every move. I studied the way he gripped the ball, the way he went into his windup, the way he followed through. What made Koufax even more of an idol was that he was a left-hander, just like me. I used to dream of throwing heat the way he did, blowing fastballs by the hitters.

After blowing hitters away like that all through college, I was drafted into the minor leagues. And for the next four years I waited, fidgeting on the threshold of my dream, just a short step away from the majors. I worked hard in the minors. Then one day I got the phone call I had waited my whole life for. I was going to the majors. The first stop was San Diego, where I pitched for the Padres. Then in 1987 San Francisco made a deal with the Padres, and I put on a Giants' uniform.

I was playing in the big leagues and being paid a big-league salary. I had a wonderful wife and two terrific kids. I was living my dream.

But then something went wrong.

Something that even my dad's big, strong hands couldn't fix.

– 2 –

End of the Dream

WHAT HELPED PREPARE me for the moment when things went wrong were a handful of memories. I've already shown you some of the memories of Dad and me in our backyard, playing catch. But I haven't shown you the ones where he's replacing the glass in the basement window after we shattered it playing ball. Or the one where he's replacing it again. And again. And again.

In all my years of growing up, my dad never put pressure on me to bear down and get serious about baseball. After all, it *was* a game. I can still hear the echo of his voice: "If it isn't fun, why play?"

I have some silly memories of him, too. In one of them he's napping on the couch after work with his shoes off. I tickle his feet and he wakes up and chases me around the house till he catches me, tickling me back till I can hardly catch my breath.

Then I can remember some late-at-night memories when he's holding me because I'm scared. I used to be afraid of monsters when I was little. Every year when the *Wizard of Oz* came on TV, I'd hide behind the couch. Remember the flying monkeys? They were the worst. Scared me to death. At night when I was in bed, I could see all the way to the folding doors

23

in the living room. And after the lights were all turned off, if I squinted a little, I could see those monkeys. Sneaking out of those folding doors. Creeping through the house. Tiptoeing their way to my bedroom. Well, that's all it took for me to throw back my covers and take off running to Dad. I'd jump in bed with him and he would put his big arms around me, holding me till I stopped shaking. And he would keep holding me till I fell asleep.

Over the past few years I've seen all sorts of things lurking in the dark. Shadowy and uncertain things. Things that frightened me. Sometimes they were coats in the closet that just looked like flying monkeys. Other times they were real, and I felt like running.

When I was a scared little kid tumbling into bed with my father, I felt peace in his strong arms. That's the same peace I felt as an adult in the arms of my heavenly Father when the coats in the closet turned out to be cancer.

It started as a small lump on my pitching arm. I didn't pay much attention to it at first. It didn't hurt. It didn't interfere with my pitching. But then it got bigger.

At the advice of the team doctor, I saw a specialist. I'll never forget that day. My wife Jan and I were in a room by ourselves, waiting for the test results. Through the door we could hear the muffled voices of the doctors.

"Look at that tumor!"

Tumor? The word hit me like a line drive. I looked at Jan. "I think we need to pray," she said.

"Dear God," I prayed, "we don't know what's happening, but whatever it is, help us get through it."

What he helped us get through was cancer. The cancer was diagnosed as a desmoid tumor, and it had to be cut out. But in cutting out the tumor, the surgeon also had to cut out much of the surrounding muscle—the deltoid muscle, the very muscle that enabled me to lift my arm and throw.

I asked the doctor how long it would take before I could pitch again. He tiptoed around the subject, careful in his choice of words. He told me I would be losing the use of the most powerful muscle in my arm. He told me that simple things like taking out my billfold would be hard. He told me I *might* be able to play catch in the backyard with my son.

Jan pressed him. "In other words, short of a miracle he will never pitch again."

"That's right," the doctor said. "Short of a miracle, he will never pitch again."

Jan and I believed in a heavenly Father with big, strong hands that could fix anything. I told the doctor, "If I never play again, I know that God has someplace else he wants me. But I'll tell you something else, Doc. I believe in a God who can do miracles. If you remove half of my deltoid muscle, that doesn't mean I'll never pitch again. If God wants me to pitch, it doesn't matter whether you remove all of the deltoid muscle. If he wants me to pitch, I'll be out there."

After surgery I went home to Ohio to recuperate. The transition from being a big-league pitcher to a small-town patient wasn't an easy one. My arm burned from the memory of the surgeon's knife. I was prepared for that. I had a prescription to push back the pain. What I wasn't prepared for was the pain that shot through me one night as I watched TV.

Jan and the kids had gone to bed. I was watching the 1988 World Series and seeing my friend Orel Hershiser pitch the game of his career. I sat there in the dark, alone with my thoughts. I couldn't help feeling sorry for myself, thinking that it could've been me out there. Instead I was sitting on a couch, alone, in the dark. And for the first time since the tumor was discovered, I cried.

In a few weeks I started physical therapy. The road to recovery was steep and strenuous, but week by week I was gaining ground. After five weeks I could take the billfold out of my back pocket. After three months the doctor was so impressed with my progress he let me go to Arizona for the last two days of spring training. There the Giants' physical therapist put me on a grueling regimen of exercises. I worked with him five days a week from April of '89 through June. He worked me so hard I felt like a prizefighter training for the heavyweight title. By midsummer my physical therapist said, "It's a miracle, but you're ready to pitch."

On August 10, 1989, I pitched my comeback game against the Cincinnati Reds. It was the highlight of my major league career. The crowd at Candlestick Park stood and cheered as I came onto the field. I couldn't believe the outpouring of love I felt that day. The scoreboard framed their feelings with the words: WELCOME BACK, DAVE!

I waved my cap to the crowd, then stepped off the mound and bowed my head to give thanks. I've never seen Candlestick Park so charged with emotion. Each inning I took the field, they cheered. It was like a dream, like the best dream you've ever dreamed in your entire life. And there I was, standing in the middle of it, a kid from Ohio, right smack in the middle of his biggest boyhood dream.

Five days after our 4–3 victory over the Reds, we traveled to Montreal. There was no stadium full of fans cheering me. There were no scoreboards welcoming me back. It was just another game as far as the Expos were concerned. Business as usual.

When I stepped onto the mound, I was ready to get down to business, too. For three innings I threw well and didn't give up a hit. I felt no pain. By the fifth inning, though, I found myself rubbing my arm. It's hard to describe the feeling. A tingling sensation. It ran halfway between my shoulder and my elbow. I asked myself if something was wrong, but I shrugged off the question. I shouldn't be surprised if my arm didn't feel quite normal. After all, my arm hadn't had quite a normal year.

The next inning my control started slipping. The first batter hit a home run off me. And *I* hit the second batter! It was an inside pitch that grazed his leg. As he walked to first base, I knew I had to come through because the next batter up represented the tying run.

Of all people, Tim Raines stepped up to bat. Tim was an all-star hitter, and I knew I had to bear down on him. Anything less and he would even up the ballgame.

I looked at my catcher, Terry Kennedy, and he signaled for a sinking fastball, low and away, on the outside part of the plate. I nodded to him and started my windup. But when I brought my arm over my shoulder, I heard a crack next to my ear. It sounded like a brittle tree limb snapping in two. It was so loud even the people in the stands heard it. The ball went sailing wildly somewhere between home plate and first base. My arm felt as if it had been chopped off with a meat-ax and went sailing along with it. Instinctively I grabbed my shoulder, but my forward momentum sent me tumbling face first to the ground, where I landed on my back. I groped for my arm, the pain knifing through it like a jagged blade. As odd as it sounds, I wasn't discouraged as I lay there, because with the excruciating pain came a strange sense of exhilaration, a sense that God wasn't finished with the story he was trying to tell with my life. It was weird. There I was gritting my teeth, biting back the pain, and I was thinking, *Okay, God, what's the next chapter gonna be?* Then suddenly I became overwhelmed at what God was doing in my life, and I realized what he was doing was much bigger than baseball.

Our first baseman Will Clark was the first to reach me. My other teammates, the coaches, the trainer, all flocked to my side. "It's broken," I said, grimacing, and they brought out a stretcher and wheeled me off the field.

Everyone knew I would be out of the lineup for a while. But my teammates were all rooting for me, even my doctor. He said the bone would heal to become even stronger because of the calcification that would build up around the break. Another comeback was certainly possible. I had done it before; I could do it again.

Or so I thought.

My arm was set and put in a brace and a sling in time for me to watch the Giants clinch the 1989 championship that sent them to the World Series. After the final pitch of that game, I ran with my teammates to the pitcher's mound and was caught in the crush of the celebration. Someone bumped me from behind, and my arm broke a second time. I was in a lot of pain and felt frustrated that I had been so careless to go out on the mound. Stupid, stupid, stupid. Why did I go out there? What was I thinking?

But a ballplayer doesn't *think* when his team wins the game that sends them to the World Series; he *reacts*. And I reacted just like the rest of my teammates.

While they were celebrating in the clubhouse over our

victory against the Chicago Cubs, I was lying on the trainer's table in tremendous pain. It was so severe that sometime later, when the World Series was delayed due to an earthquake, Jan and I decided to go home to Boardman, Ohio, for me to recuperate.

I immediately made an appointment with Dr. Bergfeld at the Cleveland Clinic. Dr. Bergfeld, the orthopedic surgeon who had originally diagnosed the tumor in 1988, was not optimistic and referred me to Dr. Muschler.

When Dr. Muschler studied the X-rays, his face grew serious. There were two distinct breaks. The bone was lining up okay, but what concerned him was a large lump that appeared just above the location of the previous tumor. On October 22, 1989, he scheduled me for an MRI, short for "Magnetic Resonance Imaging." The MRI is a diagnostic machine used to generate images of the inside of the body. It is particularly useful for spotting tumors. But the results were inconclusive, so the doctor scheduled me to come back in three months for another exam.

On the ride home from the doctor's office, the conversation Jan and I were having took a wrong turn and the road started getting bumpy.

"What are you going to do?" she asked.

"I dunno."

"Don't you think it's time to retire?"

"No," I said sharply. I had been a baseball player all my life. It was all I knew. I couldn't give it all up just like that. I couldn't just let it go. Not without a fight.

"If I were in your shoes, what would you tell *me* to do?"

"Retire," I answered coldly. I'm stubborn but I'm not stupid. I knew the facts; I just had a hard time facing them.

"Well, what are you waiting for?"

I shot her a hard glance. "It's *my* decision, not yours."
End of conversation. And start of a very quiet ride home.

Deep in my heart I knew she was right. I just couldn't admit it. I talked to a couple of old friends, Atlee Hammaker and Scott Garrelts. Both echoed Jan's advice, and I finally admitted to myself that it was time. So on November 13, 1989, I announced my retirement from baseball, the game I loved since I was seven years old.

The dream was over.

– 3 –

Beginning of a
New Journey

T HE DECISION TO RETIRE from baseball was a difficult one for me to reach. But when I did retire, I left with no regrets. Yes, my boyhood dream was over, but for me that dream was fulfilled the first day I put on spikes and suited up in a major league uniform. The rest—the all-star game I played in, the two play-offs I participated in, the World Series—was all icing on the cake. And when I came back from cancer to play again, that was the candle on the cake, the brief shining moment that flickered in the bay wind blowing across Candlestick Park on August 10, 1989.

To understand some of the stress that began to come into our lives, I'll need to take you back to the time after my comeback game on August 10 and before my retirement from baseball on November 13. It was early September. Jan and I were talking with publishers and interviewing prospective writers to work on my comeback story. We wanted the book out by spring to catch the front end of the baseball season, but we had to grease the gears to get there.

On September 5, though, those gears ground to a halt, and we found ourselves taking our first step into the wilderness.

31

We were at home in San Francisco as the team was preparing to go into the playoffs with the Cubs. I was downstairs, interviewing a prospective writer when the phone rang. Jan was upstairs with the kids and took the call. After a few minutes Tiffany and Jonathan came running downstairs to get me.

"Mommy's crying," they said.

I ran upstairs, my legs growing heavier the closer I got to the bedroom. The doorway framed Jan standing by the phone, tears streaming down her face. I tried to pick up the broken fragments of conversation to piece together what had happened. When she saw me, she handed me the phone and sank to the bed, devastated.

It was news from back home in Ohio. Bad news.

Jan's father had died.

He died suddenly at work from a massive heart attack. He was sixty-four. His death came as a total shock. He didn't have any physical problems that we knew of. He was fine the last time we talked with him.

His death had come as unexpectedly as the death of Jan's mom. She died in the bleachers of Riverfront Stadium in Cincinnati in 1982, while watching me pitch for the Padres. Also from a heart attack.

When I got off the phone, I hugged Jan and told her how sorry I was.

Jan took care of the funeral arrangements and was a source of strength to her stepmother and her brother. It was so characteristic of her. To be the strong one. To be the one to take care of the details. But there was one detail she overlooked.

She didn't grieve.

She hadn't really grieved when her mom died either. Frankly I don't think either one of us knew how.

It takes time to grieve, time to let reality settle in, time to let the memories float to the surface and do their work. But between planning the funeral, looking after the family, getting ready for the playoffs, and working on the book, there was no time.

Another reason there was no time was because our lives became very public after my comeback game on August 10, 1989. And with that territory comes a certain amount of chaos. Jan and I are not people who do well with a lot of chaos around. She's very organized and meticulous. She likes to be on top of things, to be in control.

I'm not as organized, but I do like things neat and in order. In baseball I was used to an orderly routine. On the day of a game I would have a light lunch at home and then leave for the ballpark about two-thirty or three o'clock. Once there I would get dressed and start stretching around four-twenty. After about twenty minutes of stretching I would do a little batting practice to limber up further. When I finished that, I went back to the clubhouse to relax. I wouldn't eat dinner, and around ten after seven, I'd get dressed for the game. Then I'd get by myself and pray for about ten minutes. After that I'd go to the bull pen and warm up for ten to fifteen minutes. The game would usually last from 7:35 until around 10 o'clock. Sometimes I would stay later to talk with reporters. Then I'd ice down my arm for about twenty minutes, take a shower, and head home. I'd arrive there between 11:00 and 11:30, and usually go to bed around midnight. On out-of-town games everything was taken care of for us. Someone else packed my bags. The bus came at a certain time. The plane departed at a certain time. We ate at a certain time. Everything was organized and went like clock-work.

But when I retired from baseball on November 13, I had no routine, no schedule, no one organizing my life. I was overwhelmed by the phone ringing off the wall and by the mail that came pouring in from all over the country. When I was in San Francisco, I got close to ten thousand pieces of mail. When we moved to Ohio, that figure multiplied. Our garage was stacked with boxes of mail. There wasn't even room to park the car. Jan and I became overwhelmed by just reading the mail, let alone answering it.

Besides being inundated with letters, we found ourselves swamped with all sorts of requests. Someone would ask me to speak somewhere, and I'd somehow fit it into my schedule. Someone would ask us for an interview, and we'd feel obligated to give them one. Someone would ask us to support a cause they were promoting, and we'd feel we had to say yes.

We felt pulled in four different directions. It was like being drawn and quartered by all these wonderful opportunities to do good. We just couldn't say no to people who needed our help.

To handle all the demands on our lives, Jan and I put ourselves in a go-mode. Getting the house ready for out-of-town guests. Eating on the run. Rushing to the airport. Meeting *this* person. Making *that* phone call. Answering *those* letters. Go, go, go. Our home didn't have a front door, it had a *revolving* door.

But you can only go like that for so long before it starts to take its toll. And we were digging into our emotional pockets, paying that toll, big time.

When you're under a lot of stress, you become oblivious to

the hurts of those around you. And there was someone right under our nose who was really hurting. Her name was Kristen.

Kristen was our baby-sitter, and her parents were longtime friends of ours. She was going through a traumatic time. Her parents had taken in a foster girl who was her friend, but living under the same roof together strained the relationship. Kristen felt smothered whenever she was at home. But her problems went beyond home. Her boyfriend Paul had just tried to commit suicide. He had tried several times before, but this time he almost succeeded. He was in the hospital getting his stomach pumped when Kristen's parents called. They were considering putting her in the hospital because at the time she was suicidal, too.

"Don't do that," I told them. "She can stay with us. Maybe if she was in a neutral place, it might help."

Her parents talked the idea over with Kristen's psychiatrist, who thought it was a good idea. I told Jan about the situation and about the plans I had made.

"What?" she asked, her mouth dropping open.

"God put it on my heart to help Kristen," I said. "She's moving in."

I didn't ask Jan; I told her. I didn't take her feelings into consideration or think about the amount of pressure she had been under; I just did it. Looking back, I don't know what I was thinking. I just saw a friend who needed help and figured we were the ones to give it.

Jan saw it differently.

"I COULDN'T BELIEVE Dave had invited a houseguest without asking me first, especially a houseguest who was struggling with so many personal problems. What got me so upset was that I knew where the full weight of those problems was going to land. It wasn't going to be Dave taking care of Kristen; it was going to be me.

"How could he be so sensitive to the needs of others and so insensitive to the needs of his own wife? Didn't he know what I was going through? Didn't he care?

"I loved Kristen and sincerely wanted to help her, too. I just didn't know where the energy was going to come from. I had expended it all in taking care of Dave and all the demands that had pushed their way into our lives. But I pulled up my bootstraps so I could be strong . . . one more time.

"Kristen moved in during the second week in November, a few days before Dave announced his retirement. She stayed at our house for six weeks. She cried a lot during that time. She showed me some of the songs she had written about Paul. It was obvious her feelings for him ran deep. We talked for hours on end about those feelings, about the Lord, about life. I tried to help her the best I could. I took walks with her, listened to her, sat in on meetings with her psychiatrist, encouraged her to keep a journal to help get her feelings out.

"All the while I was pushing my own feelings in. I didn't have time to deal with them. There were too many people who needed me. And they needed me to be strong.

"Tiffany and Jonathan were two of the people who needed me. For so many months I had taken care of Dave and neglected them. Now I was taking care of someone else, and once again, they were put on the back burner. I felt like a horrible mother. When caring for Kristen, I felt bad for not taking care of my own kids. When I was caring for them, I felt bad for not taking better care of Dave. And when I was taking care of him, I felt bad for not spending more time with Kristen. I was like a hamster in a cage, running around in circles in this little wire wheel of guilt. And the faster I ran, the more exhausted I got.

"Kristen left a week before Christmas. The day after she left, my brother and his family moved in to visit for the holidays. With Mom and Dad gone, he was all I had left of my family.

"Besides dealing with Kristen's problems, preparing for Christmas, and accommodating houseguests, I had to wrestle with the uncertainty about Dave's arm. Finally Dave decided that instead of waiting three months for his next MRI, he would fly to Sloan-Kettering Hospital in New York to have his arm examined by Dr. Murray Brennan, the leading authority in the country on soft-tissue tumors.

"It was late November when Dr. Brennan examined him. He studied the X-rays and the MRI, then felt Dave's arm. He was certain the tumor had returned. He wanted to operate as quickly as possible and gave us the option of scheduling surgery either before Christmas or immediately after it. Dave opted for after. Not exactly the way you want to start a new year, with more surgery and more uncertainty.

"More stress.

"More strain.

"How much *more* could Dave and I take?

"I didn't know, but I had a feeling we were getting ready to find out."

– 4 –

Surgery

THAT YEAR, getting ready for Christmas was just another thing on Jan's growing list of things to do. I could tell she wasn't looking forward to it. She went through the motions of "peace on earth, goodwill toward men," but she had no peace and her goodwill was wearing a little thin.

By the time Christmas arrived mine had worn completely out. I tried to put on a good face, but after a while I ended up retreating to my study or vegging out in front of the TV.

Her brother left on New Year's, and we left with my parents for New York two days later to check into Memorial Sloan-Kettering Hospital. Established in 1884, it was the first hospital dedicated to the exclusive treatment and cure of cancer. Our knowledge of cancer was rudimentary back then, and surgical techniques were primitive by today's standards, but thanks to generations of dedicated men and women at Sloan-Kettering, we are beginning to win the war against cancer.

Every day at the hospital the battle for human lives continues. When we arrived there, we were struck by the fact that this battle was not without its casualties. We saw them everywhere. On every floor. In every room.

I was admitted to the sixteenth floor, the gastrointestinal floor. Many of the patients on that floor were hollow-eyed, weak, and pale. They had IVs in their arm, tubes up their nose, and the shadow of death across their bed. When they moaned, their pain seemed to echo through the halls. The staff was terrific, quick to respond to their pain, but you could never get away from it—the pain, I mean—or from the harsh reality that death was just down the hall, making its rounds, working its way to your door.

Dad and Mom had made the trip with us, while my brother Frankie and his wife Missy stayed in our house and kept our kids. Together we walked down the hallway. The fluorescent squares of light were spaced evenly along the acoustical ceiling. The linoleum floor was buffed to a high-gloss finish, reflecting that light. Everywhere there was the clean smell of soap.

Not such a bad place after all, I thought to myself. Until we reached my room. The guy in the bed next to mine had a tube up his nose and was throwing up.

My mom lost it. She and Dad had been under a lot of stress, too—the stress of seeing one of their children suffer. Caught up in my own feelings, I had completely overlooked *theirs*. It was no wonder that Mom's feelings spewed out when they did. How many distraught feelings had she kept bottled up inside for her firstborn child? And for how long?

The next day, January 4, Dr. Brennan took me into the operating room. He made a T-shaped incision and found that I had extensive wounds on the remaining deltoid muscle, the muscle that extends from the shoulder and tapers into a V midway down the upper arm. He also found that the tumor had returned. He took the rest of the deltoid, leaving only a small portion intact to cover the curve of my shoulder. He also took ten percent of my triceps, the muscle on the underside of the upper arm.

To kill any remaining cancer cells Dr. Brennan, assisted by Dr. Harrison, inserted nine brachytherapy catheters.

Brachytherapy is a form of radiation treatment where thin hollow tubes, something like soda straws, are placed along the margin of tissue where the tumor was removed. Then the incision is closed, with the ends of the tubes protruding from the skin. After the wound has a few days to begin healing, iridium pellets are inserted into the tubes, which give off potent doses of radiation to kill off any cancerous cells around them that were not removed during the operation.

During recovery someone asked if I would visit the fifth floor—the children's floor. The boy I visited there was eight years old. He had had cancer since he was four. While I was there, he had to buzz the nurses for a shot of morphine to ease his intense pain. As the morphine was taking effect, we talked about baseball mostly, who his favorite player was, things like that. It was no secret who his favorite team was, with his Mets cap sitting proudly on his head.

After a while he drifted to sleep, and his mother and I talked. "As a mother," she said with tears spilling from her eyes, "you long for heaven; then his suffering would be over with."

I came away from my time with that boy and his mother with an enormous sense of sadness. I was sad that we lived in a world where suffering was so ruthlessly impartial. I longed for a world where good people were rewarded with health and happiness, where bad people were the ones who got the terminal diseases and died young. But that's not the world I found myself in as I took the quiet, hollow elevator back to the sixteenth floor.

On that floor I met a woman named Linda. She was thirty-nine and the mother of three, a boy and two girls. She had had gastric problems since the summer of 1989, and had lost a lot of weight as a result. The doctors didn't discover her tumor until Thanksgiving. By that time it was too late to operate. Instead they gave her radiation treatments and chemotherapy.

She was Catholic, and we talked a lot about the Lord. From the way she talked, I could tell she knew the Lord in a personal and intimate way. We talked about her kids and her husband, and her face lit up as she told me how much she loved them, how much they meant to her. They were all very close. She was a good woman, and she had everything to live for. But cancer is an indiscriminate disease, blind to good and evil, blind to a young boy or a mother of three.

On the first floor of Sloan-Kettering there is a mural that traces the history of the hospital. One of the quotes on the mural is from a former president of the research center, Dr. Lewis Thomas: "We are now beginning to learn how to ask very deep questions, and that is an immense step forward. The answers will come inevitably, in their own time; that side of science is the easy part. The hardest of all the tasks in research is to ask the right questions."

Early on in my battle with cancer, I discovered the importance of asking the right questions. I decided not to get mired in the question "Why." Instead I decided to ask, "What good can come out of this so that others may benefit?"

I use the word "decided" because it was a conscious choice. That choice determined my attitude. And my attitude, I think, is what helped other people I came in contact with. Seeing this fruit grow out of my own suffering kept me from being preoccupied with digging up some deep explanation for *why* I was suffering.

One benefit of suffering is that people bring all sorts of things to ease your pain. Cookies. Get well cards. Flowers. And books. Plan on receiving lots of books when you're suffering. Some of them are like Job's counselors and say a lot more than they know. Others are written by people who have had firsthand experiences with suffering and what they say is often so simple that it is profound. I received one such book written by Albert Schweitzer. Dravecky and Schweitzer. Hospital rooms bring together a lot of oddly paired roommates, don't they?

Schweitzer was a man whose doctorates in philosophy and theology equipped him to find an answer to the problem of suffering. But instead of seeking to answer it, he sought to alleviate it. After getting another doctorate—in medicine this time—he spent the rest of his life solving the problem of pain in a practical way for the natives of French Equatorial Africa. You know, I think he might have had something when he said: "Even while I was a boy at school, it was clear to me that no explanation of the evil in the world could ever satisfy me. . . . But however much concerned I was at the problem of the misery in the world, I never let myself get lost in broodings over it; I always held firmly to the thought that each one of us can do a little to bring some portion of it to an end."[1]

A remarkable thing happened when I reached out to others in that hospital in an attempt to help bring a portion of their suffering to an end—a portion of *my* suffering was brought to an end. Not the physical part, but the mental and emotional part, which is often the worst kind of suffering. The relentless throb of introspective questions. The sudden, stabbing pain of realizing the meaninglessness of your life. The dull ache of loneliness. I was spared those kinds of pain.

At least for now.

On January 10 the brachytherapy catheters were loaded with iridium pellets, where they remained for five days. During that time I was placed in total isolation. No visitors were allowed. Nobody came in except nurses, and they came in only long enough to bring me my food or administer my medication.

I had a lot of time to think. I thought about how little control I had over my life. Other people told me when to eat, when to get out of bed, when to take medicine, when to turn out the lights. I realized my life wasn't in my hands anymore. It wasn't in the doctor's hands either. My life was in God's hands. It was in his hands all along, but you don't really realize that until you see a shrouded gurney wheeled past your room on its way to the elevator.

On January 16, I said good-bye to the staff at Sloan-Kettering. I said good-bye to the boy on the fifth floor. And I said good-bye to Linda. I gave her an assignment to put on some weight. She gave me a Raggedy-Andy doll. There we were, standing in the hall, exchanging tokens of friendship like two kids at that awkward moment of departure when the one is all packed up in a moving van and ready to move to another neighborhood.

"Keep in touch," she said.

"I will," I answered, and waved good-bye.

Sometime after Linda returned home, I called to keep my promise, to keep in touch and see how she was doing. Her dad answered the phone. When he found out it was me, he started to cry. Her mother came to the phone and told me the news. Linda was dead. She had died a couple of weeks earlier. Her mother said that Linda was at peace in heaven.

After I hung up the phone, my heart was in my throat. I ached for Linda's mom and dad who were forever without a daughter. I ached for her husband who was now without a wife. I ached for her kids who would go through life without a mother.

Does a father like Linda's ever get over the death of his daughter? *Fully* get over it, I mean. Does a mother? Does a husband? A son? A daughter?

Would *my* father ever fully get over it if I died? Would my mother? Would Jonathan and Tiffany? Would Jan?

I hope not.

I hope they would eventually get over their grief and get on with their lives, but I wouldn't want them to get over me— not fully anyway. I would want to think that somewhere there was a place in their heart for just me and the memories of all I meant to them, that there was an emptiness only seeing me alive could fill, an ache only having my arms around them could satisfy, a hurt only heaven could heal.

Maybe it's selfish to think that way. But maybe not. Maybe that's how it should be. That way, with every death of someone we love, our longing for heaven grows stronger, because that is where our heart is, taken there a piece at a time by the ones we loved on this earth.

– 5 –

The First Step

DURING THE TIME after the surgery, Jan had to carry the load for both of us. And I didn't make her load any lighter. Since I liked things neat and orderly, I would get upset when I saw all the chaos in the house. To keep me from getting that way, she would stay up late at night and do everything that needed to be done.

But no matter how hard she worked, I still found reasons to get upset. I yelled a lot during the past two years. It started when I broke my arm a second time. I really hadn't been moody before that. I think it had something to do with the lack of control I had over my life.

The three C's of being a successful athlete are Confidence, Concentration, and Control. As a pitcher it was my job to control the ball, whether it was a fastball, a curve, or a slider. It was also my job to control the tempo of the game. If I was locked in a groove, I could do it, no problem. But suddenly for the first time in my life, I had no control. And it scared me. That's why I yelled, I think. The chaos at home was too painful a reminder of the chaos in my life that I couldn't control. It was as if my life were a series of wild pitches, one crazy ball after another. There was no groove to lock in to. And there was no manager to take me out of the game.

Had it been only a few weeks ago that I was so willing to give total control of my life to God? Was it "the peace of God which surpasses all understanding" that I experienced during those five days of isolation? Or was it simply the pain medication?

God had stood by me so miraculously in my comeback from cancer, but now he seemed to be withdrawing. What was he doing?

C. S. Lewis once said that God wants his children to learn to walk and must therefore take away his hand.

I don't know why I was so blind to that at the time. When raising our two children, Jan and I did the same thing. I remember Tiffany and Jonathan, still in diapers and clinging to our hands, trying to steady themselves on their feeble legs. To teach them to walk we would gradually have to withdraw our hand. Time after time they plopped down on their Pampers. But gradually they took a step on their own. Then two. Before long they were walking. Tentatively at first, but they were walking. They got a lot of bumps and bruises during that time, but they learned to walk. I wish I had read Lewis at the time. The rest of the quote would have brought me a lot of comfort: "And if only the will to walk is there He is pleased with their stumbles."

That God could be pleased with my stumbles was so foreign to my mentality as a major league pitcher. If you stumbled on the mound, it resulted in either a balk or a stolen base. Every error you committed went against your record. Every batter you walked sent your manager looking off toward the bull pen for a replacement.

"And if only the will to walk is there He is pleased with their stumbles."

Could he be pleased with me even though I couldn't perform? Even though I stumbled? Could God really love me like that?

I would spend the next two years learning the answer to that question.

– 6 –

Jan Begins to Falter

By FEBRUARY I STARTED feeling stronger. The arm was healing and with spring just around the corner, I felt a stirring sense of renewal.

Also that month we found a church to attend regularly. We had visited a lot of good churches since moving back to Ohio, but we ended up settling down in a small, non-denominational church of about 125 members.

The night of February 6, Jan and I met with Kristen and Paul. They were both seniors in high school. Paul had enlisted in the Navy and was to be stationed in Florida as soon as he graduated, but he was dreading going away. They talked to us about getting married.

We shared with them the seriousness of that commitment, what it meant for two people to become one, not just physically, but mentally, emotionally, and spiritually as well.

We talked, too, about the baggage that is brought into a relationship when two people get married. And each of them had a lot. Especially Paul.

Paul had a low self-image. He was confused and troubled. When they left that night, Paul was upset and wasn't talking to Kristen. Maybe the baggage had been too heavy. Maybe he had carried it around with him for too long. Maybe the thought of carrying somebody else's was just too much for him.

The next day Jan and I went to the 13th Annual Sports Banquet, where I was being honored as the Man-of-the-Year. It's a local deal but a pretty big one. In the past the award has been given to various sports figures like Dan Marino and Tommy Lasorda.

It was a festive evening with a few famous sports figures, among them Boom Boom Mancini, the boxer who had once been lightweight champion of the world. There were also lots of familiar faces. Two friends I had pitched with in San Francisco were there, Atlee Hammaker and Scott Garrelts. Both said a few words from the podium. Scott told me how much he loved me and that he would miss me in the clubhouse. Atlee presented me with the plaque and told the audience: "Inspiration is for a moment; a relationship with Christ is for a lifetime."

I'll never forget those words. And I'll never forget that evening—in more ways than one.

Jan and I came home late that night. Our baby-sitters, Stephanie and Amy, met us at the door. I could tell immediately that something was wrong.

"Paul's dead," they said.

"Don't tell me that," I said, the news hitting me hard and knocking me back a step.

Earlier that day Kristen had gone over to Paul's house, but he wouldn't let her in. After pounding on the door and pleading with him, he finally did. He was irrational and talked about killing himself. She talked with him for three hours, crying and begging him not to. He seemed to be doing better, and Kristen left around noon. She had called several times that afternoon to check on him. The first time was when she arrived home. No one answered. The second time was about four-thirty. A stranger answered and said that none of the family could come to the phone right now. The third time she called was around six o'clock. A policeman answered. Paul had nailed the garage door shut, started the car, and let the fumes from the tailpipe end his life.

And that night which was so warm with friendship and so glowing with accolades turned suddenly dark and cold.

The news devastated us.

"PAUL'S DEATH FELL on me like an anvil.

"Over the weeks ahead, I began to buckle under the weight of everything I had been carrying. My memory started to fade. Sometimes when talking with other people, I couldn't remember their names or what they were talking about. I felt like I was stumbling around in some dense fog where everything was hazy and muffled. Conversations seemed to float around me in wisps. I heard a few sentences, but my thoughts vaporized before I could form a reply. If you didn't know me, you would have thought I was on something, but it was stress. My system was overloaded, and it was starting to shut itself down.

"My first thought was that I was either losing my mind or else had a brain tumor. I tried to tell Dave, but he just poked fun at me. He's always had problems with his memory, so it didn't seem like such a big deal to him. But it was a big deal to me. I was scared to death, and I was afraid to tell anyone.

"In the weeks ahead I tried desperately to hold onto my sanity. I pushed myself through the motions of motherhood and routinely went about my responsibilities around the house.

I felt that if I could just hold on for a little while longer, just until our lives became normal again, I would be okay.

"But normal never came.

"It was the middle of March now, and I packed the family to fly to Washington, D.C., where Dave was to receive the American Cancer Society's Courage Award from President Bush.

"When we arrived in Washington, we were picked up and taken to our hotel. That's where I had my first panic attack. As I entered the hotel lobby, I felt light-headed. The room was spinning around, and I was afraid I was going to faint. I told Dave I needed air, and then, with my heart racing, I rushed outside. The fresh air helped and the frightening sensation left.

"But when we got in the elevator, it started again. As soon as the doors closed, fear clutched my throat. I gritted my teeth and stared down at the floor.

"'Pray for me, Dave. I'm getting dizzy.'

"'You're fine,' he said. 'Just straighten up and take a couple of deep breaths.' That's how Dave was programmed as an athlete—suck it up and get with it. If he had pain in his arm when he was on the mound, he just pitched through the pain. He sucked it up and got the job done. But I couldn't do that. I was face down on the mound. I didn't need a pep talk; I needed a stretcher.

"When we reached the room, it got worse.

"'The room's twirling around. I can't breathe,' I said as I tried to gulp air into my lungs.

"'You're just tired,' Dave said. 'Lay down and rest awhile.'"

Jan Begins to Falter

I FELT CERTAIN that after a good night's sleep Jan would bounce back. The next morning she did seem better as we all got ready to see the president.

A limo picked the four of us up and drove us to the back entrance of the White House. The grounds were meticulously kept and spring was beginning to bloom. We went through a series of sophisticated security checks and were taken to the west end of the White House. A marine in dress colors stood at the entrance, still as a mannequin. From there we were escorted to the waiting room of the Oval Office. There were no windows in the waiting room, which was filled with people waiting for their appointment with the president. It was a large room with high ceilings and beautiful paintings.

When our appointment came up, we were ushered into the president's office by some of the White House security and staff. As we greeted him, flash bulbs went off right and left. I presented him with my book and a gift from the San Francisco Giants—a Giants jersey with Bush's name and a number 2 stitched on it (his number when he played baseball at Yale). After he and the representatives from the American Cancer Society presented me with the award, the President took Tiffany and Jonathan over to his desk and showed them pictures of his grandkids.

During all this, Jan was trying to put on the best face she could. But I knew it was only a mask.

- 7 -

Face First in the Dirt

O N MARCH 29, Jan and the kids all flew with me to San Francisco where I started my book tour. But I was so busy I hardly saw them. I was making three, four, five stops a day, signing books, giving interviews, being whisked off from one appointment to the next. Half the time there I didn't know whether I was coming or going.

"I GOT LITTLE SYMPATHY from Dave when I was with him in San Francisco. At the time my heart was racing, I was dizzy, and I couldn't sleep. It was like a constant adrenaline rush.

"While Dave continued the book tour, the children and I returned to Ohio. When I arrived, I called my good friend Patty Struharik at 11:30 that night: 'I'm sick, Patty. Something's wrong with me. My body feels like it's stuck in third gear and won't stop.'

"Patty prayed with me over the phone and kept telling me not to look too far ahead. 'You're making yourself more anxious by focusing on all you have to do,' she told me. 'Just take one day at a time.'

"One day at a time, one step at a time. That's how you get

through a wilderness. If you look ahead at everything stretching before you, you'll get overwhelmed and drop in your tracks.

"On April 5, 1990, I flew to New York City to appear with Dave on a few national talk shows to promote his book *Comeback*. On the plane I had another panic attack. But it passed, and by the time we appeared on *Entertainment Tonight*, things were going better.

"That night Dave and I met with his book publicist Carol DeChant for dinner. She told me Dave's book tour would last six weeks. Well, that's all I needed to hear to push me over the edge. I couldn't hold up for another six weeks.

"The next morning when I woke up in the hotel, my heart was racing. Before we were interviewed for the *Good Morning, America* show, I sat in the makeup room, where the hairdresser was busy undoing everything I had done to my hair earlier that morning. My heart continued to pound out of control.

"When it was finally time for us to go on the set with Charlie Gibson, I said to myself, 'Dear Lord, please don't let him ask me any questions.'

"Somehow I got through the interview, and from there, we were taken to CBS. That's when the racing sensation returned. I felt if I could just get through this interview I would be okay. I had been drinking hot tea all morning, and I'm sure the caffeine compounded the problem. We got through the taping fine, but the crew had problems with the tape and had to reshoot it. By now my heart was pounding through my rib cage.

"'Take me to the hospital, Dave.'

"'What?'

"'Take me to the hospital!'

"'Now?'

" '*Now.*'

"Instead of to the hospital, he took me to the nurse's station at CBS. The nurse said my pulse was extremely fast and that I needed to see a doctor. As I lay there, though, my heart rate began to come down a little.

"Dave's publicist made arrangements to fly home with me to Pittsburgh International Airport, where Bobby and Patty Struharik met me. They took me straight from the airport to the doctor.

"The doctor said I was running a fever and had the flu. The Struhariks took me home and put me to bed. But I couldn't sleep. Late that night I called Patty. I told her I could feel myself falling apart, and I broke down crying over the phone.

"The next morning she took me back to the doctor. He felt I just needed rest. He prescribed an antidepressant, but all it did was stimulate my heart to beat even faster. I lay in bed looking down at my chest and could see my nightgown shivering in response to the pounding of my heart. I thought I was going to die.

"Monday morning I talked to the doctor again. He said I just needed to give the medication time to work. But it's hard to wait when your life is slipping away before your very eyes.

"On Tuesday night I called again, crying this time. I begged him to help me. He recommended I come in to see him again. Meanwhile I called my brother who is a pharmacist and told him what medication I was taking and how I was feeling. He said a lot of my symptoms were side effects of the drug. That scared me, and I wanted off the medication.

"On Wednesday morning Patty took me to the doctor again. He gave me a ten-question test and told me I was depressed. I denied it. I thought he was crazy. How could I be depressed? What did I have to be depressed about? I thought he just meant I was in a down mood. I knew my problem was deeper than that. I knew something was *physically* wrong. He said there was nothing else he could do and recommended a psychiatrist for me to see.

"Patty took me to see the psychiatrist, but she was livid about it. She thought a Christian had no business going to see a psychiatrist. She lectured me the whole way there, telling me that my problem was purely a spiritual battle, not a physical or emotional one.

"When we entered the waiting room to the psychiatrist's office, it seemed cold and impersonal. A sliding glass window separated the receptionist from the people who were sitting along the walls, looking at magazines.

"The psychiatrist was a fairly young man for all the framed degrees that decorated his wall. The walls of his office were painted gray. His couch was black. His coffee table was glass. Not a very cheery place for someone in the throes of depression.

"When I was in his office, I couldn't even hold my head up. I had to rest it against the arm of the chair. That's how weak I was. I told him about my side effects and what my brother had said, and he took me off the medication cold turkey.

"After the session Patty drove me home. Neither of us said a word. After she dropped me off, I called her. 'I know you're mad at me. I just needed help so badly.' But she still didn't understand how sick I was.

"Dave was in California on the book tour when I called and told him I needed him home. He could tell by my voice it was serious, and he came home that night. Just seeing him again made me feel better. But the feeling was short-lived.

"That evening was a nightmare. My body shook all over, my heart rate shot up, and I couldn't sleep.

"At 6:30 the next morning Dave called the psychiatrist and told him what I had gone through. Dave and I both went to his office. After the session I asked Dave, 'Well, what did you think?'

"'You'll never go back to that doctor again,' he said, emphatically.

"He insisted that if I got any counseling at all, it had to be *Christian* counseling. We knew of a Christian counselor in San Francisco who had helped many of Dave's teammates and their wives. As soon as we arrived home, Dave called him.

"Dave explained what had been going on with me. The counselor told him that I was going through burnout and that I needed help. He gave Dave the name of a Christian counselor in our area. He also convinced Dave to cancel the remainder of the book tour and stay home with me.

"I started seeing the counselor immediately. He also said I was burned out, both physically and emotionally, and that I needed bed rest. Because of all I had gone through the past six months, he felt I couldn't stand one more ounce of stress. He also told me I needed time to grieve over the losses that had taken place in my life.

"That was something I didn't want to hear. I didn't want to grieve; I wanted to feel better. I felt that I shouldn't be looking at the past, especially when the past made me feel so bad.

"When I shared these feelings with the pastor of our church, he told me I didn't need professional counseling. He said modern-day psychology was always having us look back on our past, but if God had given us the grace to endure hardships in the past, then we shouldn't be looking back. I was so confused. I didn't know who to believe. After three weeks of vacillating, I stopped going to counseling.

"During this time I wasn't able to function as a wife or a mother, and my guilt over that made me even more depressed. I needed help to run my home and to take care of my children. Even though I was unaware of it at the time, Patty later told me that the pastor's wife had talked with her about surrounding me with members of the church. But the presence of so many people in our home pushed away the very people we needed most—Dave's family.

"The family, for all its flaws, is God's most basic form of community. It's not a perfect community—neither is the church—but it is where we learn to care for one another. That's what families are for, to be there when you need them, to fix you chicken soup, to put fresh sheets on your bed, to get you through whatever it is you need help getting through.

"And yet our family was being kept away.

"The pastor's wife or other members of the church were at our house every day. One day I showed the pastor's wife one of the books I had been reading on depression, written by a Christian psychologist. She grabbed the book out of my hand and threw it down. 'You don't need to go to *the world* for help. All you need is the Word of God.'

"When I hear people say things like that, it makes me question whether they have really understood the Word of God, for the Word directs us to other resources outside of it. For example, it directs us to the counsel of our parents: 'My son, keep your father's commands and do not forsake your mother's teaching. Bind them upon your heart forever; fasten them around your neck. When you walk, they will guide you;

when you sleep, they will watch over you; when you awake, they will speak to you' (Prov. 6:20–22).

"It also directs us toward any people who can give us good advice: 'A man of understanding will acquire wise counsel' (Prov. 1:5, NASB). And I needed wise counsel not only from a good medical doctor but from a competent Christian psychologist as well.

"The pastor's wife continued with a smile: 'You're in God's classroom, and he's doing a mighty work in your life. Isn't that great!'

"I didn't say it at the time, but I was thinking, *No, it's not great. Who are you to speak for God, and how do you know what he's doing in my life?*

"I felt sick and alone. I had no appetite. The next morning I got up and looked at myself in the mirror. My cheeks were drawn. My eyes were sunken. The color had gone out of my face. It was like looking at someone who had literally been wandering around in a wilderness, lost and disoriented.

"I stared blankly at that stranger in the mirror. Wondering how she had gotten that way. Wondering if she would ever get better. I stared and wondered, until I could look at her no longer. On tentative legs I made my way back to bed. I closed my eyes. The image of the woman in the mirror was burned onto my eyelids.

"I could not escape her.

"And I could not escape wondering if she would make it out of this wilderness alive."

– 8 –

A Well in the Wilderness

SEEING JAN in that condition really concerned me. She had lost fifteen pounds by now—fifteen pounds she didn't need to lose. With the fixed, vacant expression on her face, she looked more like a wooden marionette than a human being.

A close friend of ours saw her one day and was shocked. He immediately made an appointment for her with an outstanding area physician, Dr. Charles McGowen. I don't know why it took someone else to step in and get Jan some good medical help, but I'm thankful he did.

"WHEN THE DOCTOR saw me, he could tell I was in desperate shape. I was living in fear. Both my parents had died unexpectedly of heart problems. I felt I was next in line.

"Dr. McGowen put his stethoscope to my chest and heard a slight clicking sound and a murmur, which he told me were characteristic of mitral valve prolapse. He explained that I had a defect in one of the valves in my heart, which was causing my heart to beat irregularly. The anxiety I had experienced caused my heart to race and compounded the problem.

"Dr. McGowen confirmed his diagnosis by doing an echo-cardiogram. After he reassured me that my condition was very common, not life threatening, and easy to prove by noninvasive testing, I started to relax. I was relieved to know that I hadn't imagined my heart problems, that they weren't just 'in my mind.' And fortunately they were treatable with medication. The doctor prescribed a beta-blocker that reduces the strength of the heart's contractions, helping to slow the heart rate and normalize irregular beats. The medication helped immediately.

"Dr. McGowen then sent me to Cleveland Clinic for further tests. The doctor there put a scope down my esophagus, which revealed that indeed I did have a very pronounced mitral valve prolapse."

D R. MCGOWEN TOLD Jan and me that the prolonged stress she had been under caused a chemical imbalance in her system. The fear she had experienced from her panic attacks caused the imbalance to become more severe, pushing her deeper and deeper into depression.

Although most people look at depression as simply emotional in nature, we learned from doctors that it is a complex condition which often has medical, chemical, and biological factors as well. These can contribute as much to a person's depression as stress, personal loss, and the influence of family backgrounds.

Depression affects different people in different ways. It can cause us to feel pain, sadness, and hopelessness. It can make us feel anxious and out of control. Worst of all, depression can cause a deep and long-lasting sense that our very soul is lost in a "black hole" that has no bottom to it. Sometimes the depressed person may even despair so deeply that he or she becomes suicidal.

Other symptoms of depression range from oversleeping to insomnia, from compulsive overeating to self-starvation, from withdrawal to frantic social activity. A person can also experience problems in logic and have difficulty concentrating.

These were some of the things Jan was experiencing.

It can be hard to treat Christians for depression, because we often think it is a spiritual problem stemming from a lack of faith. But I'm learning that many great people of faith have had devastating bouts with depression: Jeremiah, David, and Elijah, just to name a few. Elijah was even suicidal. After fleeing for his life from Jezebel, he collapsed under a tree in the desert and prayed to die (1 Kings 19:4).

When you take a look at the stress Jan had been under, it wasn't difficult to see why her system was short-circuiting. Both her parents had passed away, her mother in 1982, her father just recently. I had contracted cancer, broken my arm twice, and undergone surgery. There was the rush to get the book out. The book tour. She went through a traumatic earthquake in San Francisco in 1989, when the Giants played in the World Series. We made a major move across the country from California to Ohio. There were the problems of other people around her who needed help. Kristen's boyfriend's death. Then there was the constant pressure of the unrelenting attention that was thrust on our family because of my sudden fame. Add the fear of the return of my cancer, and it's more strain than an average person could bear. Looking back at all this, what surprises me is not that she collapsed, but that she didn't do it sooner.

Dr. McGowen's compassionate concern and his competent

medical care were like a cup of cool water to Jan's parched lips. And for the first time since her journey into the wilderness, she felt her strength coming back.

Since Jan was in good hands with Dr. McGowen, I tried to reschedule the book tour. I was also going back and forth in my mind whether I should call Dr. Brennan.

For some time now an ulcerated hole had surfaced on my upper left arm. I didn't pay much attention to it at first, because it was small. But it grew bigger, like a sinkhole. It deepened until eventually you could *see* the humerus bone. Jonathan could even stick his finger into the hole and tap on the bone, which he thought was a really neat trick.

Eventually I did call Dr. Brennan. He wanted to see me right away, so once again I flew to New York. He scheduled me for surgery to clean out the hole and repair it. But the surgery would be more involved than that. He wanted to take a muscle from my back and graft it into my arm, filling in the space left by the missing muscle.

Dr. Brennan called Jan from Sloan-Kettering, telling her I would have to have surgery again. She got hysterical and told him that I was getting ready to go back on the book tour and—

"Young lady," Dr. Brennan interrupted, "your husband's health is more important than any book tour. My job is to make sure he can go on a book tour next year, not next week."

It was hard to imagine Jan this stressed-out. She had always been the strong one, the one who had everything organized, the one who could handle anything.

– 9 –

Which Way Is Up?

ALTHOUGH JAN AND I were both in a wilderness, what she experienced in the wilderness was different from what I experienced. Because of that it was hard for me to lock-in to her pain, and hard for her to lock-in to mine.

We struggled daily in that wilderness to get our bearings. That's not an easy thing to do when you're surrounded with empty horizons, deceptive mirages, and shifting sand.

As we stumbled our way through this trackless desert, we encountered plenty of people who pointed out directions. The only problem was that we had people pointing in so many directions, we didn't know which way was up. Proverbs says that "in an abundance of counselors there is victory." There can also be confusion. Anyway, confusion is what *we* experienced with some of the counselors that came offering advice.

We had a few days before we had to go to New York for my surgery, so I took the time to read through some of the mail. The majority of mail I have received has been positive and encouraging. But a few of the letters were unsettling. They came from sincere people, I'm sure, people like the man below who just wanted to help:

Dear Dave,

I'm writing to you in hope that you'll receive the Word of God in faith and receive your *total* healing. I should have wrote you a year ago but I felt you knew the Word of Faith. Then I heard you on James Dobson and realized you were going to lose your healing by what you were saying. . . .

Dave, you could be still pitching if you don't reject this teaching and you act *immediately*. . . .

A lot of religious teachers condemn this message but praise God it works *every* time, because it's God's living Word. . . .

The Bible says ye *were* healed by Jesus' stripes. "Were" is past tense so it's already done! Jesus bore our sicknesses and diseases for us, the Bible says. Jesus healed everyone who asked it of Him while He was on earth. God's will for us is health everytime. . . .

He loves us all and He will heal any believer who has faith in what He's provided for us in His Word.

The letter quoted several Bible verses and pointed me in a direction that would lead out of the wilderness and into a promised land brimming over with health, wealth, and prosperity.

At one point in my life, getting a letter like that would have made me angry. I didn't get that way, but I did feel that the person was trespassing on private property. From spending so much time in hospitals, I've learned that when we walk through someone's door who is suffering, we have to respect the sanctity of that room. When we cross that threshold, we should be careful not to violate that person's life. Something sacred happens when a person is suffering. There is a turning to God, turning to him for assurance, for answers, for comfort.

What goes on in that room is between God and that person in the hospital bed.

I felt this man had violated that relationship when he came barging into my room. He intruded without showing me the courtesy of knocking, without even asking if he could come in. What struck me is that this guy had so many answers for my life, and he didn't even know me. He was a complete stranger, yet he was confident he had a road map from God for my life.

It seems to me that the journey of faith is not such an easy-to-follow map. It is a one-step-at-a-time kind of experience. When God called Abraham to leave his hometown and follow him, Abraham was given no map, no set of directions. He didn't even know his destination. God just said, "Get up and go to a land that I will show you."

Abraham was expected to go where God led him, a step at a time, a day at a time. There were no guarantees that the journey would be easy. He had a lot of heartache along the way, his share of danger, and the painful introspection of living with postponed hopes.

Yet he is remembered as a man of faith.

God doesn't promise us a life full of mountaintop experiences. There will be valleys to go through, too. Dark valleys. Disorienting valleys. Valleys of depression and despair. What he promises is not a road map that will give us a detour around those valleys, but that he will walk through those valleys with us.

When we emerge from those experiences, we look back and realize that that is where the growth is. It isn't on the mountaintops, above the timberline; it's in the valleys.

As I WAS TRAVELING across the country, I had another person point me in a different direction. I was in Grand Rapids, Michigan, speaking at a chapel service when I was approached by a man in his twenties. He told me I had cancer because there was sin in my life. He told me that the Holy Spirit revealed to him that God had a special plan for me—to be a preacher—but first I had to get rid of the sin.

His line of reasoning wasn't very convincing, so I asked him about some biblical characters who had undergone suffering: "What about Joseph? Was there sin in his life that kept him imprisoned for so long? Was there sin in Paul's life when he prayed three times for the thorn in his flesh to be removed and it wasn't?"

To me the issue was not whether I had sin in my life. I don't think we need any great revelation to convince us that we're sinners. The issue is not *our* character but the character of God.

Is God the kind of God who gives people tumors when they sin? Does he dole out diseases when we fail him? Say, maybe, cataracts when we lust or hardening of the arteries when we hate. Does he punish us with leukemia and muscular dystrophy and blindness?

The Pharisees thought so. When they came across a blind man, they asked Jesus, "Who sinned, this man or his parents, that he was born blind?" Jesus responded by saying "neither," and then proceeded to heal the man.

In moments of compassion like that, Jesus mirrored the picture of God revealed in Psalm 103:10–14:

> *He does not treat us as our sins deserve*
> *or repay us according to our iniquities.*
> *For as high as the heavens are above the earth,*

so great is his love for those who fear him;
as far as the east is from the west,
so far has he removed our transgressions from us.
As a father has compassion on his children,
so the Lord has compassion on those who fear him;
for he knows how we are formed,
he remembers that we are dust.

Is that the picture of a father who takes a belt to his children when they spill their milk or wet their pants? Is that the picture of a God who gives people cancer when they sin? I don't think so.

I didn't get angry with the man. I felt sad that he was carrying around such a distorted picture of God. And I wondered how that picture would get him through life when one day he would have to walk through his own valley of suffering.

ANOTHER ARM POINTING in still another direction came at me one night when I was speaking in Youngstown, Ohio, just a little ways from my hometown in Boardman. After I spoke, a woman came up to me and told me how she was once down-and-out with a drug addiction—until someone told her about Christ, and she became a Christian and was healed of her addiction. She told me that God wanted all his children to be one hundred percent healthy.

But does he? Think about that for a minute. What would God's children grow up to be like if their lives were one hundred percent healthy and happy, if all the bumps in the road ahead of them were made smooth?

Albert Schweitzer, who spent his life alleviating suffering, pondered that question:

> Look back at those hours which passed over your life so calmly and contentedly. . . . If the whole of your life had been a succession of hours like those, do you know what would have become of you? You would have become selfish, hardhearted, lonely, without regard for higher things, for the pure, for God—and you would never have felt blessedness. When did it first dawn on you that we men don't live unto ourselves? When did the blessedness of compassion bring comfort to you? In suffering. Where did your heart come close to those who were so distant and cold to you? In suffering. Where did you catch a glimpse of the higher destiny of your life? In suffering. Where did you feel God was near to you? In suffering. Where did you first realize the blessedness of having a Father in heaven? In suffering.[1]

Cancer introduced me to suffering. And suffering is what strengthened my faith. Yet that woman implied I was suffering because I didn't have *enough* faith. She seemed to be saying, Have enough faith and get the life you want. But that struck me as making God into some kind of cosmic vending machine, where, if you pushed the right button, you would get a sweet life, free of suffering.

That type of faith also denies the constructive role suffering plays in our lives. The Bible tells us to rejoice in suffering because it helps to shape our character (Rom. 5:3–4). We all want character. Few of us, though, want to go through suffering to get it—especially those of us who are Americans.

Someone once said that the difference between American Christianity and Christianity as it is practiced in the rest of the world has to do with how each views suffering. In America Christians pray for the burden of suffering to be lifted from their backs. In the rest of the world, Christians pray for stronger backs so they can bear their suffering. That may be an oversimplification, but I think there's a lot of truth to it.

The truth is we live in a fallen world, and suffering is an undeniable reality in that world. But suffering is not a very pretty sight, and illusions are a lot easier on the eyes than the reality. That's why we look away from the bag lady on the street and look to the displays in the store windows. That's why we prefer going to the movies instead of to hospitals and nursing homes. At least that's what we do in America.

Remember Linda, the woman who gave me the Raggedy Andy doll? Her death was a heavy burden for her father to bear. The burden can be shouldered, it can be shared, but it can never be eliminated. He will never be given back his daughter. Linda's children will never be given back their mother. Of course Linda's father could adopt *another* daughter. But it wouldn't be Linda. Her husband could remarry and give his children *another* mother. But it wouldn't be Linda.

Her loss will remain with them the rest of their lives.

Katherine Paterson wrote the Newbery-Award-winning children's book *Bridge to Terabithia*, a story inspired by a loss her son David had suffered. The loss was the death of his best friend, a girl named Lisa. The author describes the effect of that loss on her son:

> But he is not fully healed. Perhaps he will never be, and I am beginning to believe that this is right. How many people in their whole lifetimes have a friend who is to them what Lisa was to David? When you have had such a gift, should you ever forget it? Of course he will forget a little.

Even now he is making other friendships. His life will go on, though hers could not. And selfishly I want his pain to ease. But how can I say that I want him to "get over it," as though having loved and been loved were some sort of disease? I want the joy of knowing Lisa and the sorrow of losing her to be a part of him and to shape him into growing levels of caring and understanding, perhaps as an artist, but certainly as a person.[2]

Every loss causes some degree of suffering. The deeper the loss, the deeper the suffering. It is by the mercy of God that even in a very great loss something can be found.

And sometimes that something is your own life.

– 10 –

More Surgery

LOOKING BACK on the wilderness Jan and I went through, I am amazed that there were some things I saw with such clarity and other things which seemed as though I were in a blinding sandstorm. It was easy for me to read a letter, for example, and to evaluate it objectively and with emotional detachment. But when it came to evaluating Jan's condition, I lost all objectivity.

As I divided my time between reading mail at home and speaking on the road, my condition began to deteriorate. I experienced increased pain in my arm. I also noticed I couldn't rotate it as well as I used to. I began losing feeling in my thumb and index finger. Already I had lost several square inches of skin from the ulceration, and the surrounding area was inflamed.

I knew I needed surgery . . . and fast.

Once again Jan and I traveled to New York, this time with Bob and Patty. Dad and Mom stayed home with our kids. It was not a good trip for Jan. She was so weak I wasn't sure whether she was going to make it from the plane to the hotel.

I checked into Sloan-Kettering on May 6, 1990. While I was signing all the paperwork, Jan became dizzy. By the time we got to my room, I had her lie down in the bed while I sat on the chair. She was so immobilized she couldn't even go out to eat. Bob and Patty had to bring her food. To get her to eat they had to hold her head up.

While I was in the hospital, the Giants were in town to play New York. Several of my teammates stopped by to see me: Atlee Hammaker, Scott Garrelts, Terry Kennedy, Mark Thurmond. They looked at Jan lying in the hospital bed, and they could tell that something was wrong.

"THAT NIGHT Bob, Patty, and I left Dave at the hospital and went to our hotel. I had originally reserved two rooms, but Bob and Patty insisted we all share a room. They were worried about me and wanted to be close in case I needed them.

"And I did.

"I was lying in bed, crying. Patty was rubbing my feet, trying to relax me.

"'I don't think I have the strength to face the surgery,' I said.

"Patty tried to encourage me. 'God says he will never give us more than we can handle. His grace is sufficient.'

"Through my tears I nodded. I knew what she was saying was true, but at the time I felt too weak to handle anything.

"'What can I do for you, Jan?'

"'Read the Bible to me.'

"Patty read from Psalm 91:

> He who dwells in the shelter of the Most High
>   will rest in the shadow of the Almighty.
> He will cover you with his feathers
>   and under his wings you will find refuge.

(vv. 1, 4)

"Before long I was asleep.

"Surgery was scheduled for the morning of May 8. While in the waiting room, Bob and Patty sat with me and propped me up. I reminisced a little about Dave's career. I missed baseball. Dave and I both missed it. But at the time I don't think either of us knew how much.

"The surgery was ten hours long. Dr. Brennan cut out the ulcerated skin and cut away the damaged and inflamed muscle tissue below it. Of particular concern to Dr. Brennan was the exposed radial nerve, which is wrapped around the humerus bone. After he cleared the area, Dr. Hidalgo, a plastic surgeon, came in and assisted for the remainder of the operation.

"They worked together to remove a muscle called the *latissimus dorsi*, the wide muscle that runs diagonally from the underarm area to the lower half of the backbone. The muscle was trimmed where necessary and sutured to the biceps, triceps, and the remaining deltoid muscle to completely cover the bone and radial nerve.

"Dr. Hidalgo took some skin from Dave's thigh and grafted it on his arm to cover the exposed muscle. When the surgery was over, Dave had cuts on his back, his thigh, and his arm. He was in a lot of pain. His arm had swollen so much it looked like he had elephantiasis.

"We stayed in New York for five days, then Bob and Patty flew home with me. When we got onto the plane, it was storming at La Guardia Airport, and we had to wait on the runway for a break in the weather before we could take off. Patty sat next to me, holding my hand.

"The plane finally got off the ground, and we arrived in Ohio safely. While Dave spent the next week in the hospital recovering, I spent it in my own bed, trying to do a little recovering of my own."

WHEN JAN and the Struhariks left, I had a lot of time to think. I was surrounded by people who were trying to deal with the shattering blow of being struck by cancer. They were trying as best they could to pick up the pieces and put their lives back together.

One of them was a good-looking man in his forties who had cancer throughout his body. After his surgery he walked around the hall that circled the sixteenth floor. Fourteen laps equaled a mile. He did twenty-eight. He said he had the power to overcome his cancer, and he was determined to do it. I watched as he made those painful laps, his own private nurse following behind, carrying his IV.

As I watched I had a sinking feeling that he wasn't going to come back from cancer. I should have been encouraged by his fighting spirit. But I knew his positive attitude was ultimately just faith in himself, in his own will, his own strength. I had been far enough down the road of suffering to know that such faith brings only temporary comfort, and certainly no cure. A positive attitude can be of enormous help in combating cancer. But if that attitude stems from faith in ourselves, it's just another form of denial.

Another person on our floor was a girl who had a desmoid tumor in her calf and hamstring muscles. She was just a teenager. I visited with her and her parents. We talked baseball mostly, since they were such big fans, but during the silences in the conversation I realized something. This young, vibrant girl with her whole life stretching before her would never have the chance to enjoy the game as I had. She might not even get the chance to run the bases on a sandlot ballfield.

I saw a lot of other people on that floor, and I couldn't help thinking, *Here I am with this problem in my arm and there are people here who are going through so much more than I am. My pain and suffering is nothing compared to theirs.*

I was all alone at the hospital and wasn't sure how I was going to get home. Jan was too sick to come get me. Mom and Dad were busy taking care of her and the kids. Bob and Patty had already spent so much time up here that I hated to ask them. Asking for help is not something that comes easily to me, but I finally picked up the phone and called my agent Sealy Yates, who lives in California. After I explained to him my circumstances, he volunteered to come. I didn't even have to ask.

He caught a red-eye flight and arrived in New York a couple of days before I was released. He reached the hospital by eight that morning, tired and bleary-eyed. Boy, it was great to see him.

I can't remember any great pearls of wisdom he strung together to help me through my pain. He was just there. If I needed anything, he got it for me. It didn't matter whether it was a deli sandwich from downstairs or a pillow that needed fluffing up. He was there. He walked with me when I wanted to walk, talked with me when I wanted to talk, and prayed with me when I wanted to pray.

He slept in a rollaway bed next to mine. Several times during the night my pain would wake me up, and it was so comforting to just see him sleeping in that bed next to me, just to know that he was there.

And when we left on the private plane that my publisher so graciously furnished, he carried my bags.

Ten days after my surgery, Dr. Brennan called Jan's cousin, Dr. Mark Roh, who worked at M. D. Anderson Cancer Center in Houston. He, in turn, called Jan to relay the news. The cancer had returned, wrapping itself around my radial nerve. During surgery Dr. Brennan scraped the cancerous cells off of the nerve, but still the prognosis didn't look good—there was a chance the arm would have to be amputated. Jan asked how we would know. Her cousin told her that it would be when I began to lose the use of my arm.

When I left Sloan-Kettering, I said good-bye to the staff on the sixteenth floor, to Dennis Graham the head nurse, and to all the other nurses there. They were great. They had to be. They were the ones who had to stay behind. They were the ones in the trenches who had to dig in and continue the fight on the front lines. As for me, my tour of duty was over. I was headed for the home front.

– 11 –

Calling Out to God

B<small>Y THE TIME</small> I arrived home Mom and Dad were there with their sleeves rolled up, taking care of my whole family. I don't know what we would have done without them. Usually when Jan or I ever got sick, the one was there to reach down and pick the other one up. Not this time. We were both down this time. She couldn't help me up, and I couldn't help her. It was as though we were miles apart in the wilderness, separated by a vast, swelling sea of sand. She could see me on a distant dune, and I could see her, but that was about all we could do. We were too far apart to help each other, and too weak ourselves to do the other person any good.

Because of the recurrence of the tumor, Dr. Brennan scheduled radiation treatment for me at the Cleveland Clinic. The doctors there marked my arm with an indelible pen to map out where the target was. They lined up the target on my arm with the "bombsight" of the X-ray machine. The machine was a bulky piece of equipment. It sat upright and had an extension arm that was used to aim the X-rays. Since X-rays kill cancerous cells at a five times greater rate than they kill healthy cells, the key is to give a dose strong enough to kill the cancer without harming the surrounding cells.

It took about fifteen minutes to line everything up, but only about thirty to thirty-five seconds to do the treatment. They shot me once on the top of my arm and then once on the back, fifteen to twenty seconds on each side. The machine made a quiet hissing sound, something like a wood-burning tool. But I felt nothing, no burning, no pain.

Five days a week for eight weeks I drove to the clinic for my treatment. The trip from Boardman to Cleveland took about an hour and a half. The freeway cut through miles of rolling hills that were lush with summer foliage, a lot of oak and maple. I could almost make the drive in my sleep: Highway 224 to Route 11 to I-80 and on to Cleveland. It was a peaceful drive that eventually wound through the Shaker Heights district, an older area with stately mansions. Those drives were great for me. I'd think and pray and listen to tapes of my favorite Bible teachers. Sometimes I'd just pop in a tape of worshipful music and sing along with it. My voice wasn't exactly the "sound of music," but the hills did seem to come alive! At least they did for me.

Those eight weeks driving to and from Cleveland Clinic saved my life—my spiritual life, that is. I needed that time alone with the Lord. I needed it desperately. Maybe even more than the radiation.

In the hectic pace of the past year I had neglected to spend time cultivating the very relationship that meant the most to me. It seemed like the time had just slipped away. Now like a gift that time was being given back.

On that road to Cleveland I was starting to climb out of

the valley I had been in for so long. Unfortunately Jan was falling deeper into hers.

"As DAVE CONTINUED his radiation treatment, his spirits seemed to lift even though his body felt the effects of the radiation. He felt worn out all the time and slept a lot. Meanwhile, I couldn't feel anything. My body chemistry was out of whack and my emotions were spent. On top of all that, no one around me seemed to understand what I was going through. Until one day when a phone call came. It was a friend of Dave's who pitched with him at San Francisco. Atlee Hammaker. Atlee had seen me at the hospital and knew I was suffering. He knew because he had had a pretty rough bout with depression himself. He knew the pain, the anxiety, and that it wasn't something I could just snap out of. He shared with me about the wilderness he went through during 1985 and '86. He told me about his sluggishness and his low energy level—all things which I was experiencing. He told me not to focus on the symptoms I was experiencing, that that would just make them worse. He told me to focus on the Lord, and reassured me that my time in the wilderness would pass.

"It felt so good to know that someone else understood what I was going through. And for a while at least, his advice helped. Then the depression returned.

"Suddenly everything I had given myself to seemed so futile and fleeting. Both my parents had died, evaporating before my eyes like a retreating mirage. Dave was all I had left. Now I was in danger of losing him, too.

"I was by myself in the family room of our house when I had this argument with myself: 'What has Christianity brought me? It's brought me pain. Nothing but pain. I can't feel God. Did I ever feel him?'

"Then a wave of anger crested and came crashing down on me. I shook my fist at God. 'Don't close me out! I know you're there! Why don't you answer me?'

"I was angry because I felt I had been lied to. The road to the abundant Christian life had been pictured to me as a scenic journey, something like a yellow brick road leading to a wonderful wizard who would grant all my wishes. But where had that road taken me? It wasn't the Emerald City. And it certainly wasn't Kansas! It was more like Death Valley.

"I wanted to make a U-turn, back to the life I had before I became a Christian, back to a life that was preoccupied with material things. But when I thought of going back, I felt like the character Much-Afraid did on her spiritual journey in the allegorical book *Hinds' Feet on High Places*:

> As she looked down into the depth of the valley, the heart of Much-Afraid went numb. . . . How could one follow a person who asked so much, who demanded such impossible things, who took away everything?
>
> For one black, awful moment Much-Afraid really considered the possibility of following the Shepherd no longer, of turning back. . . . Now she could make her own choice. Her sorrow and suffering could be ended at once, and she could plan her life in the way she liked best, without the Shepherd.
>
> During that awful moment or two it seemed to Much-Afraid that she was actually looking into an abyss of horror, into an existence in which there was no Shepherd to follow or to trust or to love—no Shepherd at all, nothing but her own horrible self. Ever after, it seemed that she had looked

straight down into Hell. At the end of that moment Much-Afraid shrieked—there is no other word for it.

"Shepherd," she shrieked, "Shepherd! Shepherd! Help me! Where are you? Don't leave me!" Next instant she was clinging to him, trembling from head to foot, and sobbing over and over again, "You may do anything, Shepherd. You may ask anything—only don't let me turn back. O my Lord, don't let me leave you."[1]

JAN'S EMOTIONAL STATE was up and down a lot during the summer of 1990. But I was up, because when summer ended, so did my treatments. I had received a total of 5,000 rads of external radiation. Earlier that year with the brachytherapy I had received 7,200 rads. I was in danger of losing my arm just because of the amount of radiation it had absorbed. But the doctors were optimistic. They had had such success with this type of treatment, and we shared their optimism. Jan and I were excited that this chapter in our lives had come to an end. Finally there was hope on the horizon.

But that hope, as bright as it was, didn't dispel Jan's depression. And the cloud that hung over her got thicker and darker.

WHAT HELPED DISPEL that cloud, at least temporarily, was a vacation we took that fall. We were invited as guests of Focus on the Family to go to Montana for a restful retreat. It was the end of September, and the fall colors were beautiful. We stayed with twelve other couples at a place called Elk Canyon Ranch near Bozeman. Great food, great fellowship, and the great outdoors. What more could you want?

The restful setting and the supportive fellowship helped Jan a lot. But what should have been healing to my bones turned out to be just the opposite. At the end of our stay I started getting sick.

When we flew back to Ohio, I saw my doctor about it. I thought it was just the flu, but I didn't want to take any chances because I had a speaking engagement the next day in Fresno, California. I thought he could give me a shot or something, and I'd be on my way.

Well, Dr. McGowen took one look at my arm and knew that something besides the flu was wrong with me. It was swollen and blazing red. He took my temperature. I was running a low-grade fever, and he diagnosed me as having a staph infection.

Staph is the crabgrass of the bacteria family. It grows in clusters, spreads quickly, and is tough to root out. To make matters worse, the radiation treatments had destroyed many of the small arteries in my arm, creating pockets of infection that the antibiotic couldn't reach.

Jan and I were so discouraged. What we thought was the end of a chapter turned out to be merely a transition into a longer chapter of pain and uncertainty.

The infection had spread throughout my body. My fever shot up and my lymph glands became swollen. Dr. McGowen grounded me from going to Fresno and immediately had me admitted to Southside Hospital in Youngstown. There he put me on an IV of antibiotics to fight the infection.

After five days I was released from the hospital. I spent the next five weeks at home. The nurses tried for several days to find a good vein to plug the IV into, but so many of my veins had collapsed that they finally gave up. They ended up having to put a catheter through a vein and to install a dripline into my lower right arm.

I felt lousy. My arm was swollen, throbbing with pain, and inflamed. I was tired much of those five weeks at home, and I slept a lot. I ran a low-grade fever almost constantly, and I was anemic. On top of all that, I was tethered to a gaunt-looking IV. Like a vulture it peered down on me, constantly reminding me of my mortality.

Twice a day the nurses came to inject a shot of antibiotics into the dripline of that IV, every morning and every night. The only time I could leave the house was in the afternoon, but generally I felt too sick to go even then.

During that period of confinement, I experienced something of the isolation and loneliness that many elderly people go through who are bedridden because of some debilitating illness. I learned what it was like not to be able to walk around the block for some fresh air when you wanted it, not to be able to jump in the car and go to the store when you had a craving for something, not to be able to go to the movies when you felt bored or to a friend's house when you felt lonely.

I learned something else during that time. I started to learn how to lean on others—on my wife, my nurses, my parents, even my kids. I've never done that before. I've always been superindependent, and as a result, I've never learned *how* to ask for help. "Could you please help me?" . . . "I need you." The words sound so strange coming from my lips that it feels as if I'm saying something like, "*Hablá Español?*" or "*Sprechen Sie Deutsch?*" To me, asking for help sounded just as foreign.

Finally the doctor switched me to an oral antibiotic, which suited me fine because it freed me from the IV. Besides, I *hate* needles. I don't mind the surgeries, but I'm a baby when it comes to those needles. I took the oral medication every day for the next six months, from December of '90 to May of '91. It was a lot more convenient, but it didn't get rid of the staph. And it upset my stomach something terrible.

During that time the infection seemed to ebb and flow. Some days I would be totally sapped of energy. Other days I could feel myself gathering strength and getting better. But from one day to the next I could never predict how I would feel. Jan's health seemed to ebb and flow, too.

A hole in my arm erupted from the infection, and from that hole this yucky fluid would drain. Every day after my shower Jan would clean out the gunk that had collected there and stuff the hole with gauze strips soaked in antibiotics. Then she covered my arm and wrapped it with bandages. She did this every day for six months. My arm constantly leaked blood and fluid. It would get on my shirt, on the sheets of the bed, everywhere. But it got worse. By May the one hole had become three, and my arm was now leaking like a sieve.

Normally by May my thoughts would have turned to baseball, but not this spring. Oh, occasionally I leafed through the sports section of the newspaper or caught a game on TV, but for the most part, baseball was like a distant memory. What pushed baseball out of my thoughts was this doubleheader with cancer that had now gone into extra innings.

When cancer first came into my life, I didn't ask a lot of questions. Now I was beginning to: How long, Lord? How long will this go on? How long will I have to live with the pain, the confusion, the uncertainty?

− 12 −

Sinking Deeper into Depression

"It seemed that every time Dave started to feel better the infection would flare up again. With all the added anxiety and stress, I started sinking deeper into depression. In March of '91, a wave of depression hit me hard. I got on my knees and started praying: 'Lord, I know there is something wrong with me. I'm sinking again. Please help me, help me find out what's wrong.'

"At that time Dave was totally against me going to counseling for help, so I started praying for him, too, praying that God would somehow soften his heart. In the middle of March, when we were on vacation, I was reading a book entitled, *We Are Driven*.

"As I read, I shared tidbits from the book with him. 'I understand what's wrong with me now, Dave. I went through burnout, and then I went into depression. I know I'm a driven person. I know I'm obsessive-compulsive. I know all that; I just don't know how to get from point A to point B.'

"'If you need to get from point A to point B, then pick up your bed and walk; just do it,'" Dave said with all the bedside manner of a Marine sergeant. I couldn't understand how he could be so patient with others and yet so impatient with me. Does this happen to all men when they become husbands, or just to *my* husband?

"A month before our vacation, our good friends Bobby and Patty Struharik had sold their home and needed a place to stay. We thought it would be good for them to move in with us. It was fun for all the adults, and a lift for both Dave and me, but the two sets of children had a hard time adjusting to two sets of parents. When we returned from our vacation, Bobby and Patty decided it was best for the children's sake to move on, so they moved in with Patty's mom.

"During that time Dave and I were going through a difficult decision on whether to leave our church. Dave had had reservations about the church since the very beginning, but he agreed to attend because I felt happy there and liked the people. After about a year there, Dave was asked to be an elder. That's when his reservations resurfaced. He would come home from elders' meetings frustrated, and we would stay up till all hours hashing it out. We loved the relationships there, but we disagreed strongly with some of the teaching of the church and the way in which it was taught.

"It seemed to us as though the sermons were often aimed at specific people, and neither Dave nor I felt that was appropriate. In April, when I came home from being with Dave in Florida, the Sunday sermon was about depression. In a church of 125 members it didn't take long to figure out who the target of that sermon was. The pastor said that if you're depressed, you don't need counseling, you don't need drugs, you need to take it to the cross of Jesus.

Sinking Deeper into Depression

"If you ever wanted to see a depressed woman, you should have seen me after that sermon.

"Dave and I had a long discussion about the church. He felt torn between my feelings and his responsibilities as an elder. He was getting ready to leave for another out-of-town speaking engagement, and we really hadn't resolved the issue. But I had resolved it in my own mind. I knew I couldn't go another Sunday. Before he left I told him, 'I don't care if you stay; I'm leaving.'"

JUST BEFORE I LEFT to catch my plane, my agent and good friend Sealy Yates called. He was aware of our feelings about the church, and I relayed to him the discussion Jan and I had earlier that day. His advice to me has always been so timely and so down-to-earth. He said, "Tell her you love her and that you're in this together."

I thanked him for his advice, but when I got off the phone, I couldn't say those words. Why? I don't know. It's an emotional handicap, I think. I knew it was right to say them. I wanted to say them. But I couldn't.

Fortunately it's a long drive to the Pittsburgh Airport, and I had plenty of time to think. Fortunately, too, I have a car phone. I dialed home.

This sweet voice on the other end said hello.

"Honey," I said, "I want you to know I love you and I'm on your side. *You* are not leaving the church; *we* are leaving."

"DAVE'S WORDS MEANT so much to me. For some time now he had been learning to be sensitive to other people. Now finally

93

he was learning to be sensitive to me. When I got off the phone, I felt like a new woman. I felt that way because I knew I wasn't alone . . . and because I knew I was loved.

"The process of leaving the church was painful. Talk about stress. It felt like our guts were being ripped out. People from the church called us and asked us what was wrong. We were constantly having to explain ourselves, and the very fact that we questioned the leadership of the church put a wedge between us and many of the members.

"Suddenly then, at a time when we needed a church the most, it was gone. We had depended on our church for fellowship, for teaching, for worship, for all of our spiritual needs.

"Maybe we had depended on it too much.

"The time was right for us to leave, but when that support was taken away, we felt so alone and so hurt. What was so hurtful when we left was that we were shunned by many of our friends who remained there. Two of those were some of our very best friends, Bob and Patty. They thought we were giving up and deserting everyone, that we weren't thinking about the others in the church. Now there was not only a void where the church once was, there was this huge, gaping hole where Bob and Patty had been.

"Patty and I are total opposites. I'm tall; Patty's petite. I'm light complected; she's dark. I'm always serious; she laughs all the time. I'm organized; she's totally spontaneous. We've always laughed and said that she's Mary and I'm Martha. Our relationship has brought balance to both of our lives and a certain wholeness that's hard to describe. When that relationship was severed, it was like having a part of me die.

"Another support taken away.

"I couldn't handle the stress of leaving the church and the hurt over all those people who felt we had betrayed them.

"Everything I had depended upon, everything I had leaned on during these difficult times, everything that I looked to for support was gone. My energy was gone. My mind was gone. My church was gone. My friends were gone. And although Dave was there and trying to support me, he might as well have been in another universe for as much as he understood of what I was going through. All I had left was the Lord.

"I kept praying that he would soften Dave's heart, that he would help Dave to understand that I needed help. But whenever I brought up the subject of counseling, Dave's mind was made up: 'You can't go; you don't need it.'"

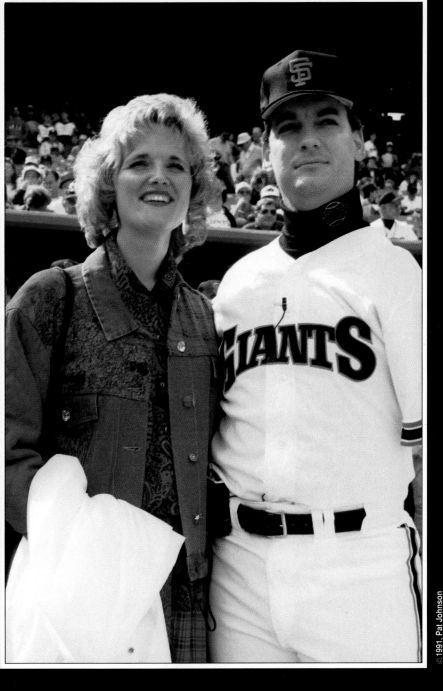

Dave Dravecky Day.
Candlestick Park.
October 5, 1991

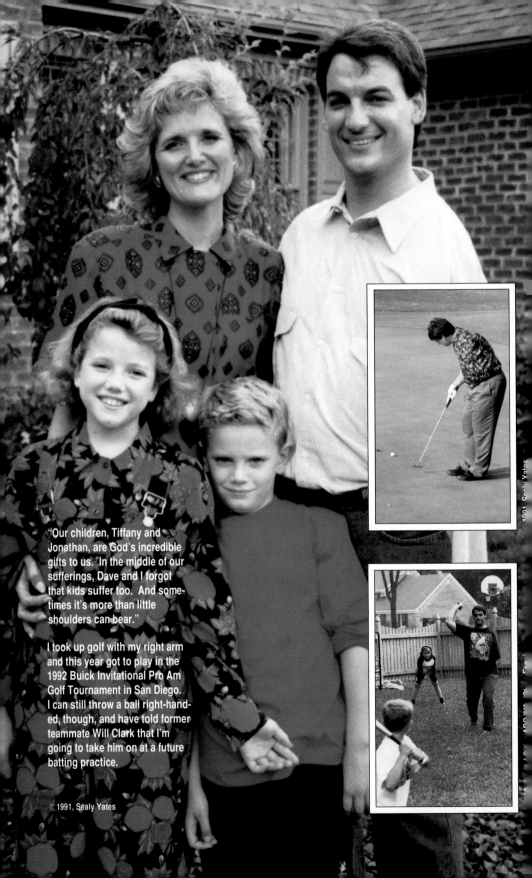

"Our children, Tiffany and Jonathan, are God's incredible gifts to us. In the middle of our sufferings, Dave and I forgot that kids suffer too. And sometimes it's more than little shoulders can bear."

I took up golf with my right arm and this year got to play in the 1992 Buick Invitational Pro Am Golf Tournament in San Diego. I can still throw a ball right-handed, though, and have told former teammate Will Clark that I'm going to take him on at a future batting practice.

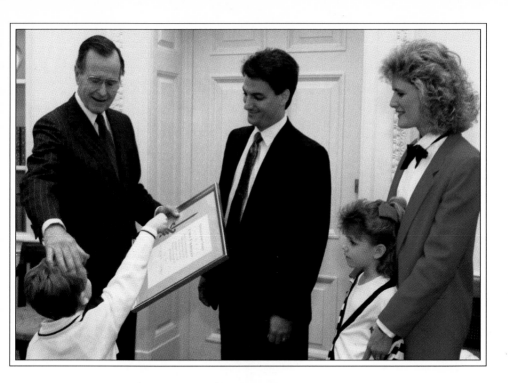

© 1991, Sealy Yates

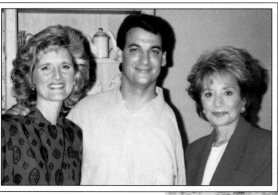

Above –"On March 22, 1990, Dave received the American Cancer Society's Courage Award from President Bush. After giving Dave the award, the President took Tiffany and Jonathan over to his desk and showed them pictures of his grandkids."

Above –"To be with Dave Dravecky is both heartwarming and heart*breaking*." Those were the words Barbara Walters used to introduce an interview that aired on ABC's 20/20, October 4, 1991.
Right–A giant get-well card from fans in San Diego.

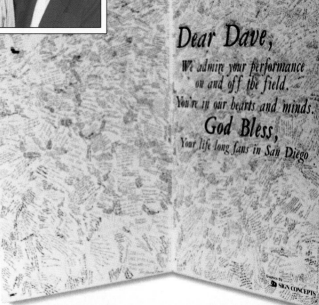

Dear Dave,

We admire your performance on and off the field. You're in our hearts and minds. God Bless,

Your life long fans in San Diego

SIGN CONCEPTS

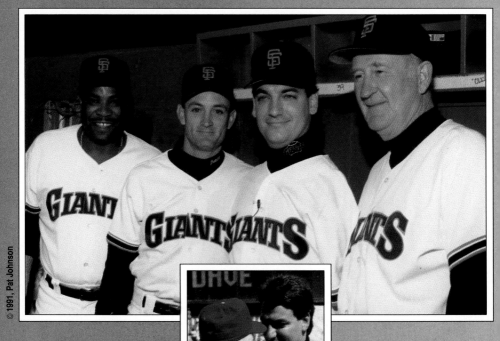

Above–Back in a San Francisco Giants' uniform on Dave Dravecky Day: left to right, Dusty Baker, hitting coach; Robbie Thompson, 2nd base; me; Roger Craig, manager. Center–The Los Angeles Dodgers were playing the Giants on that day, and it was a must-win game for Los Angeles. I spent a few minutes with Tommy Lasorda, the Dodgers' manager, before the game.

Left–First baseman Will Clark got the first hit for the Giants that day, and he belted a long ball into right field for a stand-up triple. Everyone cheered. So did I. I was a fan now.

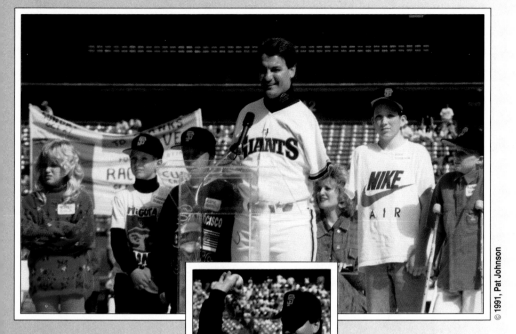

Above–During the pre-game ceremonies, the Giants gave out the "Courageous Kid Award" to five kids who faced cancer with uncommon courage: Mollie Back, Cameron Bradley, Katie Brown, Ryan Dzygunik, and Andrew Slade. They were the real heroes that day.

Center–The Giants honored me in another way that day; they let me throw out the opening pitch.

Right–I was overwhelmed with the sentiments expressed that day. I came to Candlestick Park to say thank-you. And to say good-bye. Thank-you to the Giants and the fans. Good-bye to a game I loved.

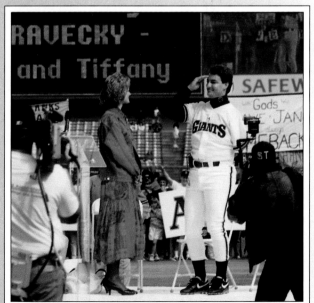

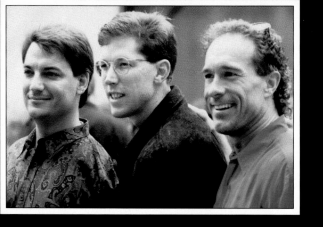

Left—I was excited about seeing old friends and coming back one more time to Candlestick. Two of those friends played for the Dodgers: Orel Hershiser, who didn't pitch that day, and Gary Carter, who caught the entire ball game.

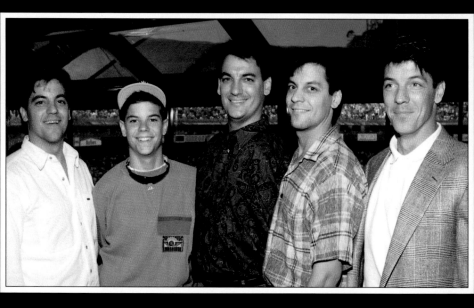

Above—My whole family came to San Francisco for this special tribute. Having my brothers around me that day made me appreciate my roots. From left to right: Frankie, George, me, Joey, Rick. Right—My parents and I had a picture taken with the owner of the Giants, Bob Lurie. From left to right: Frank Dravecky, Bob Lurie, me, Donna Dravecky.

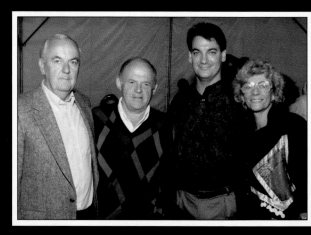

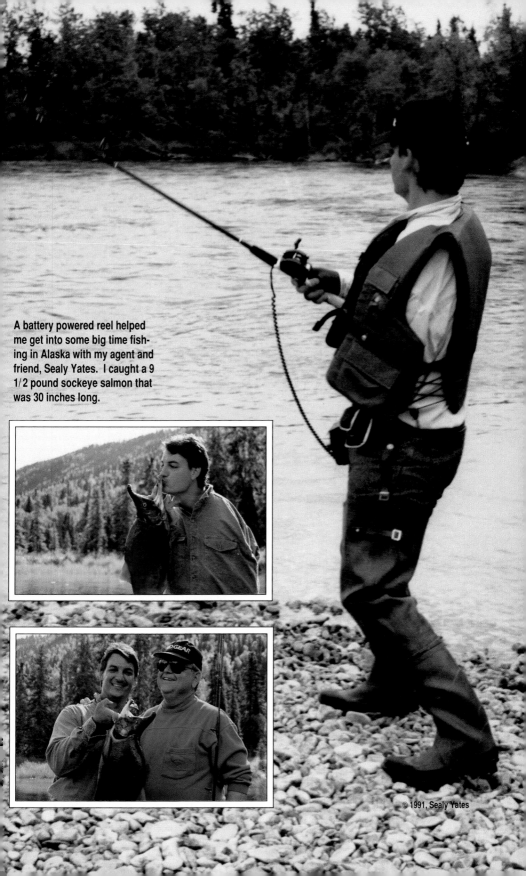

A battery powered reel helped me get into some big time fishing in Alaska with my agent and friend, Sealy Yates. I caught a 9 1/2 pound sockeye salmon that was 30 inches long.

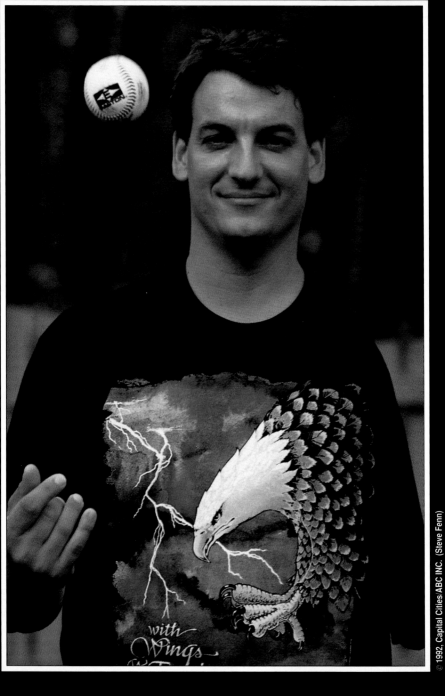

What do you do when you can't come
back? May God give you the grace to
put your hand in his–even if you have

– 13 –

The Child Who Stumbles

THESE WERE rocky times for Jan and me. We were both suffering so much with our own pain that we couldn't understand the pain the other one was going through.

When I started on the oral antibiotics, that freed me up to resume my speaking responsibilities, but I found that traveling was harder on me than before. The sustained use of the antibiotics was beginning to take its toll. And the continuing chaos around our house didn't help.

It seemed as though every time I came home from an out-of-town trip, things got more hectic at home. Without Jan organizing everything, things just piled up. My study was a mess. A landslide of mail covered my desk. Phone messages were scattered around like piles of leaves. And there were boxes of things people wanted me to sign, baseballs, baseball cards, pictures. All of this was crammed into my tiny study.

There were speaking requests, everything from a few words to a local Boy Scout troop to a motivational speech to a national business convention. There were requests for interviews, everything from the local radio station to *Nightline*. And there were requests for me to be a spokesperson for certain political causes.

I was angry with myself for not being able to do it all. And I was angry for not being able to say no.

So much of my professional life had been concerned with pleasing other people—my manager, my teammates, the fans. When I became a Christian, God seemed like just another person to please.

Could it really be true, as C. S. Lewis suggested, that if only the will to walk is there he is pleased with our stumbles? Could he love me that way, the way a father loves his toddling child?

How could he? My prayer life stank. I prayed out of desperation, not devotion. I felt I was drowning. I don't mean dangling my feet in the deep end of the pool. I mean I could feel myself going under. I called to the Lord the way Peter did when he walked on the water and started to sink: "Lord, save me!" I had so little time to pray, and when I did I felt guilty. After all, there were so many letters to answer, phone calls to return, baseball cards to sign.

So many urgent things.

A letter would request: "Please give my ten-year-old nephew a call. He's just been diagnosed as having terminal cancer and a call from you would mean so much to him."

Or a phone message on our answering machine would say: "I need to talk with you desperately, Dave. Please call right away."

Or a note would read: "My neighbor has cancer and doesn't know the Lord. If you could just talk with him, I know he would be responsive. He looks up to you so much."

I got lots of letters like that, from relatives of people who were dying of cancer or who had some terrible illness, and they were looking to me to share the gospel with their nonbelieving relatives. I was overwhelmed. First of all, I didn't even know these people. Secondly, I didn't know the depths of pain that they were experiencing.

I felt so inadequate in the face of such extreme suffering. What could I say that could possibly help them? I wanted to say, "Hey, I'm not a preacher. I'm not a psychologist. I'm just a ballplayer."

A big reason why the requests were so hard on me is that I have a hard time doing something if I can't give it one hundred percent and do it right. I knew I wasn't equal to the task. Not only couldn't I do it all, but what I could do, I couldn't do very well. And that ate my lunch.

In spite of how inadequate I felt, though, I did call many of them. And I think they genuinely appreciated that I did. All most of them wanted was to share their story of suffering with someone who would listen, someone who cared.

And I could do that.

Even a *ballplayer* could do *that*.

But the requests mounted into the hundreds, and soon I became overwhelmed. I became that way because I *genuinely* wanted to help each and every person who contacted me. But at that time in my life I had nothing to give. My tanks were all empty. I was running on fumes.

I think that's also why I was so irritable with Jan. I had tried to be Solomon for so many people that when I was with Jan I didn't want to be Solomon anymore. I wanted to be just Dave. I didn't want to think about any deep questions or solve anybody's personal problems or be responsible for any life-changing decisions. I just wanted to coast into my driveway, turn off the motor, and park myself somewhere.

One of the reasons Jan and I had nothing to give each other was that we had both been too busy. We had been so busy with urgent things that we had neglected the important things, like time with the Lord, time with our kids, time with each other. There just didn't seem to be enough hours in the day. Our calendar was booked. But even so, when something else urgent came up, we would ink it into our schedule.

A big part of the problem was me. I tried to do everything myself, to be a one-man team. I don't know why I felt that way, because even when I was on the mound, I had eight other guys backing me up. And there were plenty more in the dugout in case any of us needed relief.

Another one of my problems was that I kept trying to keep score with God, just as I did when I was a ballplayer. To a professional baseball player, everything is tied to performance. Your batting average. Runs batted in. Number of errors. For a pitcher your ERA was the main statistic everyone looked at. The letters stand for Earned Run Average. It means the average number of runs you allow to score in nine innings. So if your ERA is three, that means on an average you let the opposing team score three runs in the course of a game. The lower the pitcher's ERA, the better chance his team has of winning. If I went nine innings and gave up a minimal number of hits, no walks, and maybe one or two runs, my manager and teammates would give me a pat on the back and acknowledge my performance. But all of a sudden, there was no scoreboard, no manager to pat me on the back and let me know how I was doing.

But *I* knew I wasn't doing well. And I was so angry with myself.

But the person I took it out on was Jan.

It all came to a head on Friday, April 19, 1991. I'll never forget that day. I was supposed to speak that night to the youth group at Youngstown Baptist Church, but I felt like such a hypocrite. Here I was getting ready to tell a bunch of teenagers how to make Christ the center of their life, when he wasn't the center of *my* life; he was buried somewhere under the mountain of mail.

We were in my study when my anger vented: "How can I share Christ with them when I don't have time to spend with him myself?"

"Don't worry," Jan said, trying to ease my frustration. "You'll do fine."

"Don't worry," I snapped back. Then in a rage I swept all the letters off my desk. "I'm sick of this! I'm done! Finished! I can't do this anymore!"

I was sick and tired of it all. Tired of the pedestal people had put me on and tired of being in the spotlight and expected to inspire people every time I spoke.

I felt lousy that night. But I went. And I spoke. I felt so unworthy to be standing there in front of all those people that looked up to me. If they just knew what I was really like, what thoughts went through my head, what words came out my mouth, they'd get up and walk out the door.

But when I finished speaking, they didn't walk out. Instead one of the men in the church came forward. He was a thirty-four-year-old welder. He had been having an affair with another woman but was in the process of trying to put his marriage back together. He wanted Christ to come into his heart and change his life.

He went home that night a different person. In the weeks that followed, everyone around him noticed the change, people in the neighborhood, at work. No one noticed more than his wife.

Five weeks later that man went to get a tool from the toolbox on his flatbed truck when another truck backed into him, crushing his chest. He died instantly.

Later, when I was speaking on a nationally broadcast radio program, during the call-in segment of the show, his wife called in. She told me that those five weeks were the best days of their marriage. Choking back the tears, she thanked me.

Me, the hypocrite.

Me, the guy who was done, finished, who couldn't do this anymore.

Me . . . the child who stumbles.

– 14 –

The Turning Point

By THE BEGINNING of May, I was traveling all over the country, speaking and making public appearances. All the while I was struggling with the staph infection, the nausea from the antibiotics, and the incessant pain.

In May we also found another church. When Jan shared about her depression with the wife of one of the associate pastors there, she told us how her husband had suffered from depression, too. In fact, his was so severe he had to be hospitalized. He had been admitted to the Minirth-Meier Clinic and was successfully treated. We also learned that the senior pastor's wife used to work at the Minirth-Meier Clinic in Dallas.

They said Jan needed help and that it was not only okay to seek counseling, it was biblical. They quoted the verses about "bearing one another's burdens" and how "in an abundance of counselors there is victory." But after an earful of this, I was still skeptical.

As May wore on, my arm was beginning to wear out. So was my patience with Jan. I didn't care what the new pastors thought, counseling was for emotional wimps. It was weak to be open, transparent, and vulnerable. It was strong to hold everything inside. Anyway that's how I dealt with *my* problems. The attitude I had when I faced struggles was the same attitude I had as an athlete: Suck it up!

One day when Jan was feeling down, she told me she needed help. I thought all she needed was to get alone with God and work out her problems one-on-one.

"What do you need help for? Christ is sufficient to meet all your needs, isn't he? The Bible is adequate to answer all your questions, isn't it?"

I told her it was a lack of faith to go to a psychologist, that it was worldly, that it was a sign of weakness, that it was wrong—all things I had heard in our former church.

"I'm sick, David. I need help."

"Then go see the pastor!" I yelled.

"I need *professional* help!"

I got so angry I threw the portable phone against the wall.

"A BROKEN PHONE. What a striking image of everything that was wrong with our relationship. No matter how long I cried, Dave wasn't getting my message.

"Maybe he could keep me from going to counseling, but he didn't say I couldn't get counseling from a book. I retreated to the bookstore, where I browsed around in the psychology section. I picked up a book by Dr. Henry Cloud, a psychologist and co-director of the Minirth-Meier Clinic in Newport Beach, California. The book, now titled *Changes That Heal*, described four critical decisions that could bring hope and direction in a person's life. One of those decisions was setting boundaries. Boundaries—boy, did he have me pegged in that chapter. One reason I had collapsed was that I wanted to do everything for everybody. I felt it was my responsibility to help anyone who came to me with a need. *Anyone.* And it almost destroyed me. The book confirmed to me that I really did need professional help.

"In mid-May I accompanied Dave to California to do a taping session with Dr. James Dobson and Focus on the Family. When Dave's agent Sealy Yates met us at the airport, he told me he had a book he wanted me to read by a new client of his. It was the book by Dr. Henry Cloud that I had picked up at the bookstore. My mouth dropped.

"'You mean Dr. Henry Cloud is your client?' I couldn't believe it.

"'Yes,' he said.

"'Do you think you could make an appointment for us? If I could just speak to him to find out what he thought, even if it was just on the phone.'

"While Sealy was busy trying to set up an appointment, Dave and I did our interview with Dr. James Dobson. He asked how we were doing, and we told him how much we had been through and how bad we were hurting. Dr. Dobson sat with tears in his eyes as we told him our story.

"Then he shared how his father had gone through a similar experience with depression. His father was thirty-nine at the time and a preacher, a tired, burned-out preacher. He had driven himself to exhaustion and couldn't preach for two years.

"As he told us about his father, it was like he was telling my story all over again. I knew how his father felt. I had walked in those shoes. I had cried those same tears."

When You Can't Come Back

THE NEXT DAY as a favor to a friend, Jan and I stopped by Orangethorpe Elementary School in Fullerton to speak to about sixty kids, ranging in age from kindergartners to third graders.

I showed them a video of some of the footage of my comeback game and from the game in Montreal where I broke my arm. I explained my surgeries to them, and they all listened intently, asking a lot of questions about where the doctor cut me, how long the scar was, things like that. I asked them if they wanted to see the scar, and they got all wide-eyed with excitement. Show and tell.

I could hardly lift my arm at that point, so Jan had to help me take my shirt off. I told them that when my back itches I can scratch the back muscle that had been sewn into my arm, and the itching would go away. They all thought that was pretty amazing.

When I finished, the kids flocked around us with scraps of paper for me to sign. A few of them who had known I was coming had baseball cards; one even had a baseball. Signing my name was about all I could do with my arm at that point. As I pushed my hand through the loops and curves of my name, the words of Dr. Brennan came back to me, leaning on my shoulder, whispering in my ear: "It's time."

"As IT TURNED OUT, Sealy wasn't able to get Dave and I together with Dr. Cloud. But he was able to set up an informal visit with his partner, Dr. John Townsend. As a favor to Sealy, Dr. Townsend very graciously gave us two-and-a-half hours of his Sunday afternoon. It was a beautiful time. He made us both feel so relaxed.

"After listening to some of my struggles and hearing my symptoms, he said: 'Janice, you're off the charts as far as stress points are concerned. Do you know that?'

"'Doctor, I'm not even done yet.' And I proceeded to tell him everything else that had taken place.

"He looked at us both with his jaw hanging open. 'You know, the two of you, it's unbelievable that you're still married.'

"'Why?' we both answered.

"'Well, both of you are working with such deficits, and you're both hurting. It's just amazing that you're still together.' He told us I was suffering from burnout that led to my depression. He said I could well be physically sick.

"Then he turned to Dave and said, 'Your wife needs help and she needs it now, and I'm sorry to tell you this, but as much as you love her, you're not the cure-all.' We learned that Dave's denial of my sickness came from a sense of shame and guilt he had over my being depressed. He felt my depression was a reflection of his failure as a husband. Of course, it wasn't. It didn't have anything to do with that. But Dave felt it did. That's why he got mad so much whenever I told him I needed help. Getting mad is what he did to keep from feeling like a failure.

"To my surprise when Dr. Townsend finished, Dave softened. 'Okay, John, what do we have to do?' It was the first time Dave realized how sick I was.

"Dr. Townsend then helped find someone in our area that could help me. He referred us to Dr. Lorin Sommers in Canton, Ohio, a little over an hour from where we live.

"That was the beginning of my healing. And that was the beginning of my realizing just how much God loved Jan Dravecky.

"He had caught me just in time.

"I wondered: How could I have ever experienced God catching me if it weren't for the free-fall that led me to his arms? And how could I have ever experienced the free-fall without the bottom dropping out of my life?"

– 15 –

Getting Ready to Go to New York

At ABOUT THE TIME Jan and I found a good Christian psychologist to go to, we were feeling this enormous ache in our hearts for Bob and Patty. We missed them so much. For some time now we sensed the relationship was growing farther and farther apart. Jan and I finally decided to call them to talk about it. I called Bob, and the four of us went out for coffee. I told them we felt as though we had the bubonic plague the way everyone from the church was avoiding us. I told them that just because we left the church didn't mean we left them.

At first Bob was quiet. Jan and I then shared our reservations about the church. They said they had some of the same reservations, too. We told them we feared they had been harboring hurt feelings against us. They told us they feared *we* had been harboring hurt feelings against *them*. Once we got those fears out in the open and realized none of us had any hurt feelings toward each other, the wall between us came down. It was such a wonderful time of healing. Amazing, isn't it, the medicine that's in a cup of coffee and a few honest, heartfelt words?

One by one, God was giving back everything that the wilderness had taken away. He gave Jan back her physical and emotional health by leading her to Dr. McGowen, Dr. Townsend, and Dr. Sommers. He gave us another church to attend and a whole new group of supportive friendships. And he gave us back Bob and Patty.

But there was one last thing the wilderness would take away before we left it, something that would never be given back.

ON JUNE 7, I FLEW to New York for my three-month checkup. My arm was almost immobile. I could move it only at the elbow, and then only about twenty degrees. My shoulder was extremely sore. I experienced a few sharp pains, but most of the time it was a dull ache. It wasn't so much the pain that bothered me as the lack of mobility. All I could do was write, but to do even that I had to pick the arm up with my right hand and place it on the table. It was as though the muscles had lost their memory and forgotten how to move.

Dr. Brennan came to the conclusion that it looked like it was time to amputate.

Up to this point I had hoped for the best, but I had prepared for the worst. Still the news was hard to take. I think it was hardest for my mom. Thirty-five years earlier she had given birth to a healthy baby boy—two arms, two legs, ten fingers and toes. Now she had to stand by helplessly as surgeons removed one of those arms. Her son would be handicapped the rest of his life. Both my parents tried to hide their anguish, but I could tell it hurt. I know how much it would have hurt me to see Jonathan or Tiffany face a similar fate.

Getting Ready to Go to New York

Dr. Brennan wanted to operate as soon as possible. He scheduled surgery for June 18, 1991.

The Giants issued a press release that announced my surgery. As soon as the news hit the media, our phone didn't stop ringing. I was speaking at a business convention in Michigan at the time, so Jan was the one who had to field the phone calls and visitors. One of those visitors came the day before we went to New York.

"IT WAS SATURDAY and I was frantically rushing around the house, trying to get everybody packed before Dave and I left for New York. I was packing the kids' clothes at the time. They were going to stay with Dave's brother Frankie and his wife, Missy. I bounced back and forth between their suitcases and the telephone like a Ping-Pong ball. Back and forth, back and forth. It was driving me crazy. A lot of people called to give advice about healing: 'Do this; don't do that. Believe this way; don't believe that way. Drink this; don't eat that. Pray, fast, repent, believe, tithe.' One prescription after another.

"After a particularly exhausting phone call, I got on the floor and threw a temper tantrum right in front of the fireplace.

"'It can't be this hard, Lord. Please, please, take away the confusion.'

"I picked up my Bible, and it fell open to Hebrews 12. The verse that caught my eye was, 'Endure hardship as discipline.' *As* discipline. It didn't say hardship *was* discipline. It didn't say God was bending us over the bed and beating our backsides to get us to straighten up. It said to endure hardship the same way you would endure your parents' discipline. And how do we do that? By submitting to it and enduring it.

"I skimmed through the passage and stopped at verse 11: 'No discipline seems pleasant at the time, but painful. Later on, however, it produces a harvest of righteousness and peace for those who have been trained by it.'

"Peace. That's what I needed. That's what I so desperately longed for. I realized then that peace *would* come, but that it would come *later*, as the *fruit* of my struggle, as the *harvest* of a long growing season. What I needed until that harvest was a farmer's patience.

"I actually felt a little bit of that peace, but only a little bit and only for a little while. It wasn't long before the phone rang again. And again. And again. With each interruption I got more worked up about all I needed to get done before we left.

"Then at five o'clock the doorbell rang. 'Who on earth could *that* be?' I grumbled to myself. I marched to the door with my fist clenched and my eyes glaring. I pulled open the door, and there stood this stranger, a man in his thirties.

"'You don't know me, ma'am,' he said, 'but I'm from Cleveland and I have the gift of healing.'

"I looked into his eyes. This was a man on a mission. And it *wasn't* to help me with my packing. My heart sank.

"'Your husband just needs more faith,' he said.

"I leaned against the brick wall, thinking, *God, I can't handle this.*

"'I've had cancer twice,' he explained, 'and I've been healed. Ma'am, I'm here to tell you that your husband doesn't *have* to have his arm amputated.'

"That's when I started to cry. And when I started to cry, I lost it, I mean, completely lost it. I jumped on him like a pit bull on a postman. 'I'll tell *you* something! My husband may not be perfect, but he loves God and he has faith! Tell me why there's suffering in the Bible, will you? Why wasn't Paul spared from suffering? Didn't *he* have enough faith? And how about Job? And . . . and . . . and Joseph? What about them? Huh? Did *they* lack faith? Is that why *they* suffered?'

"The man burst into tears.

Oh, no, I thought to myself, *not a crying man on my front porch. Please, God, not this.*

"'I–I'm sorry, Mrs. Dravecky,' the man stammered through his tears. 'I'm, eh, new at this thing' . . . (more crying) . . . 'I just wanted to help. I prayed to God when I was diagnosed with Hodgkin's disease, and he healed me' . . . (sobbing profusely now) . . . 'then God brought it back. I don't know why, but he brought it back. I don't understand it. The second time I prayed about it, I was led to take radiation treatments.'

"While he was crying, I was thinking to myself: *If God healed him, why did the cancer come back? And why would God heal him the first time cancer appeared and then lead him to radiation treatment the second time?* My heart went out to the man; he was more confused than I was. I put my arm around him and tried to be of some comfort as I walked him to his car.

"'Thank you, Mrs. Dravecky. And I'm sorry I bothered you.'

"'That's all right. I appreciate your concern.'

"I went back inside and plopped on the couch, thinking, *What a day!*

"The next day was Father's Day. Bob and Patty had arranged a prayer service. Two pastors from two different churches spoke. Dave's mom and dad were there, along with brothers Rickie, Frankie, Joey, and their wives, and Dave's teenage brother, George. We sang, we prayed. It was beautiful.

And it was just what we needed, to be surrounded so lovingly by our family and our friends.

"Dave and I prayed that during his stay in the hospital God would open doors to people's hearts, using our circumstances in some way to bring them comfort. Dave especially hoped for an opportunity to pray for the doctors and nurses before they operated on him.

"Later we drove to Pittsburgh Airport through the quiet countryside with its rolling meadows and its slender trees yawning toward the sky. It is hill country along the border between Ohio and Pennsylvania. Quaint farmhouses. Weathered wood barns. An occasional deer. We passed a sprawling mine on the right, black with mounds of coal, its smokestacks billowing white. A muddy river curved around it, slow and unhurried.

"The landscape we traveled through was a perfect picture of the landscape of our hearts.

"It was a peaceful ride."

– 16 –

The Decision to Amputate

JUNE 17 I CHECKED into Sloan-Kettering Hospital. A Monday. After I was admitted, Jan and I took the elevator to the sixteenth floor. My parents were with us, along with Bob and Patty and my brother Frankie. It wasn't foreboding at all. In fact, it was kind of like old home week, a lot of high-fives and slaps on the back.

"Hey, Dave."

"How ya doin', Dave?"

"Good to see you again," they said, but then they caught themselves. "Of course, not under these conditions."

Later that afternoon after we got settled in my room, Dad started crying. There was something he wanted to tell me, but the words had to be brought up from the depths of his heart. And bringing them up wasn't easy.

"I'm so tired of seeing you in so much pain, son, with that dead limb hanging from your body. . . . Just get it off and be done with it."

Telling me that was the hardest thing I think my father had ever done. Mom was real quiet, off to the side. It was too painful for her to say it, but she knew he was right.

When I met with Dr. Brennan, he told me that there was

115

an outside chance the arm could be saved . . . if there were no signs of the tumor . . . if he could correct a few things. Of course he wouldn't know until he got in there and got a good look around. He was cautious about taking the arm. He wanted the surgery to be exploratory, then give me a couple of days to think about my options.

I told him I didn't need a couple of days. I was ready for it to come off. But he told me, "I just can't do that."

That night after everyone left I watched TV for a little while, then fell asleep. A nurse woke me up at 6:00 A.M. to take a shower and get cleaned up. Jan, my parents, my brother Frankie, Bob and Patty, they were all there in the room. The mood was very upbeat, although Mom was still quiet.

Around noon I was put on a stainless steel gurney with its freshly washed green sheets and its neatly tucked hospital corners. Before I was wheeled off, I said good-bye to everyone. My parents gave me a hug and a kiss.

I picked up my left arm with my hand and waved it, jokingly, "Bye-bye, everybody."

Jan accompanied me down the elevator. Sterile, antiseptic smells mingled in the air as the elevator opened to surgery. There was a waiting area outside the operating room where the nurse parked me. Jan and I were both peaceful. As I lay on my back with the white glare of fluorescent lights in my eyes, I felt God's presence, that he was in control.

A nurse came by to ask me if I was allergic to any drugs and injected the anesthesia into the tube of my IV. That was at about twelve forty-five. I don't remember anything after that. It's all a blank.

The Decision to Amputate

"I KISSED DAVE and waved good-bye as the nurse wheeled him into the operating room. In the waiting room I sat with Dave's parents, Frankie, Bob and Patty, along with several other friends.

"We knew the surgery would take several hours, so Dave's parents left the hospital for a while to get off by themselves. They had both grown up in the Catholic Church. Dave's mom had lost her mother when she was five and was raised by Slovak nuns since the fifth grade. She and Dad Dravecky walked the summer streets of Manhattan, and between First and Second Avenue they found a little Catholic church. They went inside to pray. Their prayers, I found out later, were simple requests, almost childlike expressions of love and gratitude: 'Dear God, please let him be healthy, and thank you for keeping him alive.'

"An hour passed, and Dave's parents returned. We sat in the waiting room, thinking, talking, praying, silently hoping for a miracle. Maybe when they got in there they could do something—improve the circulation, cut out the infected tissue, something. We hoped for the best. We hoped for a miracle. God had done it before in Dave's life. He could certainly do it again.

"Two hours passed. Then three.

"Around four o'clock a nurse came out. She brought no news of a miracle. Instead she told us they were going ahead with the amputation.

"We had known all along that this was more than a possibility, that it was a probability. We were prepared for that, as well as we could be anyway. We tried to hold back the emotion, at least until the nurse left. When she did, we all hugged each other and cried together for about ten minutes.

"Dave's dad finally broke the silence: 'If God could send his

117

son to die, and all that he's asking for is my son's arm, then I can live with that.'

"At 5:10 the nurse came out and told us the operation was over. Dave was resting in recovery.

"At 6:30 Dr. Brennan came out and talked with us. He said he had to cut back into the healthy tissue to make sure he had gotten all the cancer. He said what Dave needed most was a lot of rest. He also said that in spite of Dave's faith and buoyant attitude about losing the arm, that he would have his 'down' time, a time when he would grieve. It's a natural thing for amputees, he said, and a very healthy thing.

"Dave's parents and I left the group in the waiting room and slipped in to see Dave. We tiptoed across the squares of polished linoleum so as not to wake any of the other patients. Stopping at his bed, we looked at him lying there.

"We were horrified at what we saw.

"Dr. Brennan had told us the night before what kind of procedure he would perform if he couldn't save the arm. He had even come back at ten o'clock that night to go over it again. He told Dave what his body would look like after the surgery and talked about the types of artificial limbs that were available. Dave was as prepared as he could have been. But for Dave's mom and for me, the reality of amputation hadn't sunk in.

"Until now.

"I looked at her and could tell she was angry. I love Dave as much as a wife could love a husband. But I could never love him the way his mother does. I could never know the depth of her feelings, those maternal instincts that naturally want to protect. How she must have hurt when she saw her little boy lying there in that bed.

"Dave's mother shares a history with him that I can only

share through her recollected stories. She remembers the first word he spoke as a baby; it was the word 'ball.' She remembers the winters when Dave would sit in the family room and throw a tennis ball against the brick fireplace, so anxious for spring to arrive so he could go outside and play baseball. She remembers when spring would come and how he would take his ball and glove everywhere he went. She remembers the Little League games and how even then he talked about playing professionally. She has so many feelings going on inside, feelings only a mother could know. I could not blame her for being angry. I might have felt the same way had it been Jonathan.

"As I looked at Dave's pasty, postoperative complexion, I wondered how *he* would take it when he would first see himself in the mirror. Dave has remarkable courage, but still I wondered. . . ."

AFTER I WOKE UP in recovery, the first thing I felt was how parched my mouth and throat were. The first thing I heard was the sound of moaning from the patients on either side of me. I looked at the foot of my bed and saw two hazy figures standing there. Were they angels? My eyes came into focus. Almost angels. They were Jan and my mom. And when I blinked my eyes a few times, Dad came into focus. Jan came alongside the bed and put her hand on my forehead. I was a little cold after surgery, and her hand felt warm and soothing as it brushed across my brow.

The next sensation I felt was hunger. I hadn't eaten since the day before, and I was famished. All I got, though, was a Q-tip dipped in lemon juice to suck on. Two hundred dollars a day for a room, and when you call room service, they send you a Q-tip! Sheesh! What I needed was a couple of burgers, some fries, and a chocolate malt.

Dream on, Dravecky.

They did upgrade me to a better room, though. At about nine o'clock that night they moved me to the sixteenth floor. Room 1638. I lifted my head off the pillow and tried to sit up and take a look around. Wrong thing to do. My head started to pound, and I gingerly placed it back on my pillow.

The next day I tried to get out of bed. I started feeling a little queasy so I lay back down. Then I caught my breath and went to the bathroom. That's where I saw myself for the first time since the surgery, in that little bathroom mirror. I stood there pale and rumpled in my hospital gown, staring at the image that stared back at me—the image of a one-armed man.

I was shocked at how radically they had cut the arm back. The incision started at my neck and went in a diagonal to my underarm area. The arm was gone. The shoulder was gone. The shoulder blade was gone. And the left side of my collar bone was gone.

"Okay, God. This is what I've got to live with. Put this behind me; let me go forward."

And when the one-armed man looked back at me, there was peace in his eyes.

I cleaned myself up a little and took a walk down the hall. The nurse who had administered the anesthesia stopped me.

"I really appreciated your prayer," she said.

I took a step back. "What prayer?" I asked.

"You prayed this beautiful prayer for the doctors and the staff. In fact, you prayed twice."

I was totally blown away. It was one of the things I really

wanted to do before I went under, but I had no memory of my doing it. None.

Then she went on to say, "I've heard a lot of people praying for loved ones as they go into surgery, but that was the first time anyone has ever prayed for us."

A couple of days later Dr. Brennan was making his rounds, followed by about six interns and fellows. He took the gauze off my wound and checked the incision, the stitches, the drain. It was a brief visit. When he and the others left, one of them stayed behind. A man named Jim. He told me his parents were missionaries in Mexico. He commented on my prayer in the operating room and how peace seemed to permeate the room.

At that point I realized God had granted me the desire of my heart—to pray for the medical team that would perform the amputation. He let me do it in spite of the anesthesia.

A couple of days later when I was walking around, pushing my IV, I came to the visitors' room down the hall. An entire family was huddled there, sitting, waiting, paging mindlessly through last month's magazines on the coffee table. I sat down next to the mother. Her husband had cancer throughout his body, and his prognosis wasn't good. You could tell they were all taking it hard.

I asked how she was doing. "I'm okay," she said. But I knew she wasn't. She was hurting. You could read the worry between the lines on her face.

Her son sat down beside me and asked: "Where do you get your peace?"

He had seen me in the halls, talking to several of the patients and their families, and could tell that cancer hadn't shattered my life. I could still smile and laugh. He knew something was different about me, but he didn't know what. I think that's what prompted the question.

I told him that Jesus Christ was the source of my peace. The entire family listened as I shared my faith. When I was finished, the woman said: "But, you know, my husband has never done anything bad. He's worked hard, been a good husband, a good father—yet he's in here with cancer while all sorts of bad people are out on the streets, healthy."

It's hard to understand the suffering in this life, I told her, but this much I did know: You can't blame God for it. Sooner or later our life on this earth is going to pass. Even the best lives someday come to an end. The only thing that will matter then is whether or not we'll get to heaven. I believe in miracles, that God can and does heal people, but more importantly than that, I believe in the eternal hope of heaven. When I die, that's where I'm going, because heaven is my home.

The family was quiet. I didn't know whether they believed what I said or whether they were just being polite. I went back to my room and got a copy of my book *Comeback*. I recommended she read the last two chapters to her husband.

"It tells about the hope I have in my relationship with the Lord," I explained.

Pat Richie, the chapel coordinator for the San Francisco Giants, had flown to New York to be with Jan and me, and I asked him if he would visit the woman's husband. He spent about thirty minutes with him before the man was wheeled into intensive care. He was bleeding internally, and the doctors couldn't stop it.

On the day Jan and I were leaving, both of the man's sons came into my room. They told us their father had died. We expressed our sympathy, and then the oldest asked for me to pray for their mother.

"Okay, I'll pray for her," I said, thinking I would do it later.

The oldest one looked me in the eye. "No, now."

He dropped to his knees, and his younger brother who was standing beside him did the same. It was a sacred moment. And as they knelt, I bowed my head and prayed.

– 17 –

Coming Home

Ever since that backyard game of catch with my dad, baseball had become my life. It's what I watched on TV when I was indoors. It's what I played when I went outdoors. It's what I read about when I sprawled on the living room floor and spread out the Sunday paper.

My life was wrapped up in baseball. And my life as a ballplayer was wrapped up in my arm. It wasn't long before that arm gained the attention of the neighborhood. When they chose up sides for sandlot ball, I was the one they all wanted on their team.

They wanted me for one reason—my arm.

It wasn't long before that arm caught the attention of the entire school, when, as a teenager, I pitched my first no-hitter. My name started showing up on the sports page. Before long it made the headlines.

All because of my arm.

That arm attracted the attention of major league scouts, and the part of me that was my boyhood became my livelihood. My ability to provide for my family was not based on how good of a personality I had, how smart I was, or how hard I worked. It was based solely on what my arm could do on game day. The more strikes that arm could throw, the more I was worth. The more games that arm won, the more people wanted me on their team.

When people talked with me, it was the center of conversation. "How's the arm today, Dave?" . . . "Is your arm ready for tonight?" . . . "Better get some ice on that arm; don't want it to swell."

My arm was to me what hands are to a concert pianist, what legs are to a ballerina, what feet are to a marathon runner. It's what people cheered me for, what they paid their hard-earned money to see. It's what made me valuable, what gave me worth, at least in the eyes of the world.

Then suddenly my arm was gone.

How much of me went with it? How much of what people thought of me went with it?

I don't know. But I do know this. I should have grieved over the loss of my arm. It would have been the natural thing to do. It would have been the healthy thing. But I didn't. Instead I had a cavalier attitude about it. I joked around before surgery and waved the arm in the air, playing like it was saying good-bye to everyone. After surgery I called out to my friend Bob: "Maybe now I can get a decent parking space; ya know, in one of those handicapped spaces."

My humor was a form of denial. I was afraid to face how I really felt about losing my arm. All the people I had been so critical of for denying reality—the faith healers, the positive thinkers, the sunshine-all-the-time Christians—how was I any different from them?

In time, my grief would surface. But for now, I buried it deep inside where nobody could see it; so deep not even I could see it.

Coming Home

There was a sense in which it was a relief to have the arm amputated. I had been in such pain over the past year, and all the medication and radiation had done a number on me. I was so weak and weary from it all that having the arm taken off was like dropping a heavy backpack after a twenty-five-mile hike. I felt better immediately.

I also felt apprehensive. I wondered how my son would react when he saw me. Would he be afraid? Would he feel sorry for me? Would he keep his distance? And what about my daughter? Would she be embarrassed when we went out to eat? How would she feel when people stared? How would my wife feel? What would she think about a man who couldn't tie his own shoes? Would she still find me attractive, or would she be repulsed to see me in my nakedness with my carved-up body?

When I came home from the hospital, I realized that all Jonathan wanted was to wrestle with me and play football on the lawn. All Tiffany wanted was to hug me. All Jan wanted was to have her husband back.

They didn't care whether I had an arm or not.

As important as it had been to my boyhood, as important as it had been to my livelihood, my arm meant nothing to the people in my life who mattered the most. It was enough that I was alive and that I was home.

– 18 –

Living as an Amputee

I HAD A LOT of adjustments to make as an amputee. One positive adjustment—I didn't have to listen anymore to people hassling me about being a lefty!

Everything I do now I do with my right hand. I eat with my right hand, brush my teeth with my right hand, write with my right hand. I was surprised how quickly I adapted, especially to writing. And it surprised me I didn't get more frustrated than I did in switching over.

I found I can do pretty much everything I did before; it just takes me longer, that's all. I still can't tie a tie, though. I've learned the steps to take to do it; I just haven't mastered the technique. I get around the tie thing by not wearing suits. When I go somewhere to speak, instead of wearing a coat and tie like I used to, I just wear a pair of slacks and an open shirt instead. And when I have to fly to get there, I try to just carry one bag.

I usually wear loafers and boots instead of tie shoes. And whenever I wear tennis shoes, I have these clips that I put on the shoestrings. That way I don't have to tie them; I just pull the clips tight.

Eating is something I have to take a little more time doing.

I guess that's good because I used to inhale my food. Mom was always after me to eat slower. It's a little tough cutting a steak with just one hand, but I have a special utensil at home called a rocker knife that enables me to do it.

You wouldn't think something as simple as putting toothpaste on your toothbrush would be an adjustment, but it was. If the toothbrush is flat, it's no problem. But if it's contoured, it can be a challenge because the toothbrush falls over on its side a lot when you're putting on the toothpaste.

I try to stay away from button-down collars and button-up Levis. Buttons are pretty awkward to deal with when you've just got one hand. Reading is also harder to do with one hand, trying to hold the book, to turn the pages, and my reading has suffered as a result.

I try to do as much as I can for myself, although there are a few things Jan helps me out with. Every now and then she tucks in my shirt when it starts to creep out of my pants. And when we're at a restaurant, she'll cut my meat. I'm an independent person by nature, so one of the adjustments of living as an amputee was learning to depend on other people. But still I miss being able to do things with my own two hands. During that summer I also realized that I missed something else—baseball.

There is a scene in the movie *Field of Dreams* where Shoeless Joe Jackson—one of the eight White Sox players who were banned from baseball for conspiring together to lose the 1919 World Series—said this: "Getting thrown out of baseball was like having a part of me amputated. I've heard that old men wake up scratching their legs that have been duffed for fifty years. I'd wake up at night, smell of the ballpark in my nose, feel of the grass on my feet. . . . Man, I loved this game. I'd have played for food money. It was the sounds, the smells. Ever held a glove to your face? I'd have played for nuthin'."

That scene had a powerful effect on me. Having my arm amputated and also having baseball lopped off from my life, I knew exactly how Shoeless Joe felt. I missed those feelings, too, missed the smells, the sounds. The feel of stitched seams as you cradle a new ball in your hand. The smell of seasoned leather as you bring your glove to your face. The sound of a bat cracking out a base hit.

I'd have played for food money.

I'd have played for nuthin'.

Up to this point I hadn't really missed baseball. But now that my arm was amputated, I started to. Maybe it was a kind of phantom pain from the part of me that was severed. I don't know, but I could feel a burning sensation where baseball had once been.

There are times when I watch a game on TV that I'll put myself in the pitcher's place, mentally going through the motions: the quick look to the base runner, the windup, the pitch, the follow-through. One time I even had a dream about it, a dream so vivid I was sure it was real. My arm had somehow grown back. I don't remember who I was pitching for or who I was pitching against; I just know that it was me out there on that mound. I was pitching again, and it was the most exhilarating feeling.

My grief for being cut off from baseball was beginning to work its way to the surface. It was painful. It wasn't a sharp pain; more like a dull ache. And for the first time since my retirement I admitted to myself that I missed the game.

I missed the competition, the battle between me and the hitter. I missed the part of the game where the catcher and I worked out the game plan together. I think of the times Terry Kennedy and I worked on those plans when we played for the Giants. I think of the special bond we had, of the chemistry that was there. When I got into a groove, I felt locked-in with T. K. It was an incredible feeling of oneness, two minds melding into one. I miss that. I miss it more than I ever realized I would.

Not seeing those guys on a daily basis; I miss that, too. Not being able to spend time together anymore. I think of some of the guys I played minor league ball with: Dan Gausepohl, center fielder; Jerry DeSimone, second baseman; Ron Meridith, pitcher; Mark Thurmond, pitcher. We all came to know Christ about the same time, around 1981 in Amarillo, Texas. They were such good friends.

I think of Eric Show who pitched for the San Diego Padres when I was there. I think of how he challenged me in my faith when I was just a baby Christian, still wet behind the ears. I miss being challenged like that. I also miss Thurmond from my San Diego days. What a good friend.

I think of my days in San Francisco, and Atlee Hammaker and Scott Garrelts come to mind. They were both pitchers and both would give you the shirt off their back. I appreciated their honesty, their integrity, their faith, and what fun they were to be around. Atlee and his wife Jenny. Scott and his wife Kathy. Jan and I spent a lot of time with them, doing things together as families. We used to see each other almost every day. Now it's maybe once or twice a year.

I miss those times. I miss those relationships.

Sometimes I feel the burning all the way down to my fingertips.

– 19 –

Kids Suffer, Too

"DAVE HEALED fairly quickly after the amputation. Before long he was giving interviews, making public appearances, answering letters, back to his old routine.

"One evening he took a break in that routine and took us all out to dinner. While we were eating, a stranger came by the table offering his condolences, chatting a minute, and wishing Dave the best. A few minutes later another stranger came by and asked for his autograph.

"When he left, Tiffany turned to Dave and said: 'Daddy, why don't you change your name to Smith or something and get a fake arm so you can be just like all the other dads and be at home with us.'

"It was her way of saying, 'I need more time with you, Daddy.'

"Over the past two and a half years, Dave and I had been on a hectic schedule. It was difficult for us, but the real ones who paid the price were the kids. Even before cancer came into our lives, Dave's schedule made him an absentee father during the baseball season. He would get up after they went to school, leave for the ballpark before they got home, and come home from the game after they were already in bed. When the team was on the road, he'd be gone ten to twelve days at a time.

"As an athlete Dave was constantly leaving, always saying good-bye. I realized that went with the territory of being a ballplayer's wife. I could understand that. The children couldn't. They missed their daddy. They needed him to be there, for a sense of security if nothing else. It didn't make any difference whether he was puttering around in the garage or parked behind the newspaper; they just needed to know that he was there for them if they needed him.

"When Dave retired from baseball, he changed caps but his routine remained essentially the same. He would kiss us good-bye and be gone a week at a time, traveling from city to city just as he did as a ballplayer.

"The kids missed Dave as a ballplayer; they missed him just as much after he retired.

"During the past two and a half years, Jonathan and Tiffany would fight with each other, pout, throw temper tantrums, put their toes over the lines we drew for them. It frustrated us when they acted like that. Because we had been gone so much, we felt guilty when we disciplined them. But then we felt guilty when we didn't. For a long time we didn't know what was going on. We didn't know if it was just a phase they were going through or if we needed to read more books on raising kids or what.

"It finally dawned on us that they were just trying to get our attention. It was their way of saying, 'Hey, Mom. Hey, Dad. We miss you. We need you. We're hurting, too.'

"I knew they were hurting one day in September of '91, when Dave was on the road. I was supposed to fly to San Diego to spend a few days with him there. It would have been the first time I had left the kids since Dave's amputation on June 18.

"As I was tucking them in bed, they started to cry. Real tears, not spoiled cries. This happened on a Monday night. I finally got them calmed down, and they went to sleep. Tuesday night the same thing happened. They both were hysterical, burying their heads in their pillows and crying, 'Don't leave. Please don't leave.'

"'Why are you kids putting up such a fuss?'

"'Because we don't want you to go,' sobbed Tiffany.

"'Why?'

"Through her tears Tiffany explained, 'Because if anything happened to you and Dad, I wouldn't want to live. How could you stand to have your parents die, Mom?'

"So that was it. For most children death is a vague, faraway thing that they don't think about much. For Tiffany and Jonathan it wasn't. The death of my dad had affected both of them more deeply than I realized. My mind went back to a recent family vacation in Florida. There was a big thunderstorm over the Gulf. Jonathan and I were looking at the lightning. He was quiet as he watched the jagged light rip through the black, coastal sky.

"'What's wrong?' I asked.

"'I was just thinkin'.' His voice cracked when he said it, and a tear fell from his eye.

"'Why are you crying?'

"'I was thinkin' about Papa Roh.'

"Papa Roh was what he and Tiffany called my dad.

"'Papa Roh?' I asked. 'What made you think of Papa Roh?'

"He took the back of his hand and wiped his cheek. 'I was

just wonderin' about the lightning, if Papa Roh was sending it down from heaven, and it made me think of him and miss him.'

"Suddenly Tiffany started crying, too.

"We talked a lot about Papa Roh that night. Flashes of him streaked across Jonathan and Tiffany's memory and lit up their faces: how he used to blow on their arms, how he always had bubble gum for them, how he kidded around and played with them.

"Remembering that night helped me console the kids. They weren't afraid of being alone for a few days. They were afraid of being alone forever. They were afraid I would die.

"The next morning I called Dave, explained what had happened, and asked if I could take the kids with me. I woke the kids up and told them to pack their bags.

"Tiffany's eyes widened. 'You're taking us?'

"The kids looked at each other and shouted, 'Yippee!'

"Dave and I had suffered for so long that we forgot something. Kids suffer, too. In different ways. To different degrees. But their suffering is real. And sometimes it's more than little shoulders can bear."

– 20 –

"Why Does God Make You Suffer?"

"To be with Dave Dravecky is both heartwarming and heart*breaking*." Those were the words Barbara Walters used to introduce an interview that aired on *20/20*, October 4, 1991.

A number of people wrote to tell me how much they enjoyed that interview. As I read those letters and reflected on that day the *20/20* crew descended on our house, I couldn't help but to see the disparity between image and reality. People commented how poised I looked, how relaxed and at ease I was. That was how I appeared. You want to know how I really was? I'll tell you.

Jan and I had gotten up extra early that morning to prepare for the arrival of the crew. The New York camera crew drove from their hotel in Pittsburgh and arrived around eight-thirty. They were a really great group. They spent the morning arranging the lighting, rearranging the furniture, setting the camera angles, getting everything just right before Barbara arrived.

Our family and friends had come to witness the event and

were all milling around like extras on the back lot of a studio, waiting for the director to arrive and start filming. The chaos that resulted from our house being turned into a studio was distracting. Further distracting me were the cluster headaches I was experiencing. I took some pain pills, but they didn't do a lot of good.

When Barbara arrived, she was polite but very professional. Once the interview started, I could sense her getting locked-in. She had such control, such finesse. I think I admired that most about her because that's what I was like when I got on the mound. I was a finesse pitcher. I didn't have any one pitch that would blow a batter away. Instead I depended on my knowledge of the batter and my ability to control how he would swing. I'd lull him off balance with a few pitches and then throw one low and inside, just barely over the plate. Swing and a miss.

Barbara asked me several questions, all of which I had answered sometime or somewhere before: "What came into your mind when you heard the word tumor?" . . . "What did you feel like when the arm was off?"

Every time she lobbed me a question, I took a swing and got a pretty good piece of it. Then she threw me a curve: "Why does God make you suffer?"

It caught me totally off balance. I hesitated a second then started to take a swing at it: "So I can give people that hope. . . ." But I cut short my answer and told her honestly: "Good question, Barbara."

Haltingly I tried to follow through with an answer: "I don't focus on 'Why me?' but what good can come out of it and how I can help others."

Swing and a miss.

"Why Does God Make You Suffer?"

I don't think she was trying to throw one past me. I think she really wanted me to step up to the plate and knock that one out of the ballpark. But I hit nothing but air.

Since then I've had a lot of time to think about that question. I've asked it over and over again: Why does God make us suffer? *Does* he make us suffer? I've received letters from people who think he does.

One of those letters came from a woman who aspired to be a national champion skater. Two weeks before the finals, a wheel fell off her skate and she tore up her ankle. She had numerous operations and tried to make a heroic comeback, but her ankle just wouldn't let her. She can no longer move her ankle from side to side and can't play any sports anymore. After she became a Christian, she looked back on her suffering and had this to say: "I was picked to have this pain so I could eventually be born again in Christ."

Another letter came from a man who had lost his wife of forty-seven years to leukemia: "*Why her?* I asked. But I came to realize she was chosen to suffer beyond what most humans experience, and in so doing, demonstrate a quiet faith that was a sublime example of the relation of a Christian to God."

Another letter came from a person who had lived with epilepsy since she was sixteen. She wrote: "I believe it's just something God has given me to deal with. I truly believe that I would not appreciate my life as much without it."

Did God pick out that skater and cause her ankle to break? Did he choose that man's wife to suffer beyond most human experience? Did he give epilepsy to the one woman when she was sixteen years old?

Jesus said, "Are not two sparrows sold for a cent? Yet not one of them falls to the ground apart from the Father's will." By saying that, is Jesus implying that God is the cause of the sparrow's death? Is he saying that God sits in heaven and says, "Okay, it's time for that pigeon with its nest on Second Avenue to die," and then puts the poor bird in the cross hairs of his rifle and squeezes the trigger?

Sounds silly when we put it like that, doesn't it? But that is what people imply when they say God picked them to have pain or chose them to suffer or gave them a disease.

So why do people say things like that about God?

When great pain comes into our lives, it's devastating. When C. S. Lewis lost his wife to cancer, for example, he said his faith collapsed "like a house of cards." When it did, he questioned God's character: "Not that I am (I think) in much danger of ceasing to believe in God. The real danger is of coming to believe such dreadful things about Him. The conclusion I dread is not, 'So, there's no God after all,' but, 'So this is what God's really like.'"[1]

When suffering crashes into our lives, we have a hard time understanding how a good and powerful God can be at the helm of the universe. Didn't he see it coming? Couldn't he have steered clear of it? Didn't he know how much pain it would cause? Didn't he care?

We fear asking such questions because we may come "to believe such dreadful things about Him." We fear coming to the conclusion: "So this is what God's really like."

To protect God's character from the assaults of such questions, we look for ways to explain the suffering. We may look to ourselves, saying the suffering came because we deserved it, because our sin was so great or our faith was so small. Or we may look to a higher good, saying that the benefits derived from the suffering outweigh the pain inflicted by it.

If you look at the three letters, that's exactly what the writers do; they look for the higher good. Aren't the skater's broken ankle and broken dreams small things to exchange for eternal life? Doesn't the lasting example set for others by the woman dying of leukemia outweigh the temporary pain of her death? Isn't epilepsy a small price to pay for a true appreciation of life?

I believe the problem here is that these people are confusing the *result* of their suffering with the *purpose* of their suffering. Let me give you an example.

When I went back to see Dr. Brennan for a checkup, I asked him what they did with my arm after they amputated it. I didn't want to take it home and have it bronzed or mounted on the wall or anything like that; I was just curious. He said it was sent to the pathology department and was sectioned for research.

As a *result* of my surgery, the hospital got a specimen it could study to advance its knowledge of cancer. That's a good thing, because what they learn will be used to help others with the disease. It wouldn't be such a good thing, though, if the *purpose* of my surgery was to provide an arm so that the pathology department would have a specimen to study. If a doctor performed an unnecessary amputation on a healthy person, even for a purpose as noble as medical research, he would be ruled a sadistic butcher by the hospital board and lose his license. And yet we indict God as being that kind of surgeon when we confuse the results of our suffering with its purpose.

One of my favorite passages in the Bible is 2 Corinthians 1:3–4. "Praise be to the God and Father of our Lord Jesus Christ, the Father of compassion and the God of all comfort, who comforts us in all our troubles." If we turn things around and say that the good which comes out of our suffering is the reason for our suffering, we confuse something more than results and purpose. We confuse the character of God and turn things around there, too. He then becomes not the Father of all compassion but the Father of all chastisement; not the God of all comfort but the God of all trouble, who troubles us in our comfort. That's why our understanding of suffering is so important. It affects how we view God. And how we view God affects every area of our life, from how we worship to how we raise our children.

God willed a world that is as mysterious as it is majestic. I believe God rules over that world, but I don't believe he gave me cancer. He allowed it. Why? I don't know. I don't know the purpose of my suffering. But I do know the results. When I compare the Dave Dravecky before cancer and the Dave Dravecky after, there's no comparison.

I used to see everything in black and white; now I see the shades of gray in between. I used to be dogmatic and think there was an answer for everything; now I realize a lot of things don't have answers. I used to think I could put God in a box; now I believe his ways are too deep for any box to contain. I used to depend on myself; now I depend more on God. I used to be preoccupied with my own needs; now I am learning compassion for the needs of others. I used to view Christ's death on the cross intellectually; now I view it more emotionally. Through my own suffering I have become more aware of his. And I love him more as a result.

"Why does God make you suffer?"

Good question, Barbara. A very good question.

– 21 –

The Questions That Suffering Raises

W
HEN SUFFERING STRIKES, we don't need an interviewer to frame the questions for us. Suffering does a pretty good job of that all by itself. Over the past three years, I've had a number of people send me some of the questions their suffering has raised.

A young man sent this one: "I worked so hard and prayed so hard to get into Stanford. I felt confident he would get me in, but then the door shut in my face. I was so hurt. If God is all-powerful, why did he let me down so hard?"

A girl with a rare and painful skin disease asked this one: "I often wonder why God had to give me this problem. I mean, why not a drug addict or someone like that? Why an innocent girl just trying to get through life without too many hurts?"

A twenty-three-year-old woman from Baltimore shared this question: "I am not a religious person. My parents never took me to church. I am an only child and last month my father died. He was supposed to live long enough to see me get married and see his grandchildren. I keep asking myself, 'Why did *my* dad have to die?'"

When I first learned I had cancer, I did not ask, "Why me, God?" But don't get the wrong impression. It isn't bad to ask that question. The Bible is full of people who, at some time or another, couldn't make sense of life and came to God with their questions: "Your hands shaped me and made me. Will you now turn and destroy me?" (Job 10:8); "If I have sinned, what have I done to you, O watcher of men? Why have you made me your target? Have I become a burden to you?" (Job 7:20); "How long must I wrestle with my thoughts and every day have sorrow in my heart? How long will my enemy triumph over me?" (Ps. 13:2).

Those questions were asked by Job and David, great men of faith. David is referred to in the Bible as "a man after God's own heart." Job is described by God himself as "righteous and blameless; there's no one like him on the entire earth." And yet they came to God asking some very strong, straightforward questions.

There is no such thing as a bad question. The issue is not with the questions we ask, or even how we ask them. The issue is where we go with our questions. Any question that brings us to God for an answer is a good question. Anytime we come to God, it is an act of faith. When we knock on heaven's door, regardless how hard we knock or how long we knock, how stubbornly or how angrily, we state by our very presence at that door that we believe God is there, that he is in charge of the world, and therefore in some way responsible for what goes on here.

One day a letter arrived in our mailbox, and it contained some very pointed and forthright questions:

The Questions That Suffering Raises

Dear Mr. Dravecky,

If there is a God who cares so much for you, why did he allow you to have the surgery in the first place? I have lived 41 years in this old world and I have yet to see any piece of genuine evidence that there is anything real about any religious beliefs. God certainly does not love me and has never done one single thing to express love to me. I have fought hard for everything I have in life. Nobody cares about what happens to me and I don't care much what happens to anyone else either. Can't you see the truth that religion is nothing but a crutch used by a lot of weaklings who can't face reality and that the church is nothing but a bunch of hypocrites who care nothing for one another and whose "faith" extends not to their actions or daily lives but is nothing more than a bunch of empty phrases spouted off to impress others?

My son would have been thirteen years old next month. He died at two-and-a-half months of age from crib death. How can there be a god of any sort when such unfair, horrible things happen every day? What have you got to say about that Mr. Dravecky? Is a senseless, cruel tragedy the act of this loving God you supposedly believe in?

I appreciate the man's frankness. His questions are honest questions. I appreciate that, too.

And so, what does Mr. Dravecky have to say about those questions?

I wish I could answer them, but I can't. I cannot pretend to know how that man feels or understand how the pain of that loss has shaped his view of life, of God, of himself. I can only share the experience of another father who also lost a son. The son was twenty-five when he fell to his death in a mountain-climbing accident. The father struggled desperately to make sense of his suffering:

> I cannot fit it all together by saying, "He did it," but neither can I do so by saying, "There was nothing he could do about it." I cannot fit it together at all. I can only, with Job, endure. I do not know why God did not prevent Eric's death. To live without the answer is precarious. It is hard to keep one's footing.
>
> Job's friends tried out on him their answer. "God did it, Job; he was the agent of your children's death. He did it because of some wickedness in you; he did it to punish you. Nothing indeed in your public life would seem to merit such retribution; it must then be something in your private inner life. Tell us what it is, Job. Confess."
>
> The writer of Job refuses to say that God views the lives and deaths of children as cats-o-nine-tails with which to lacerate parents.
>
> I have no explanation. I can do nothing else than endure in the face of this deepest and most painful of mysteries. . . . To the most agonized question I have ever asked I do not know the answer. . . . I do not know why God would watch me wounded. I cannot even guess.
>
> . . . My wound is an unanswered question. The wounds of all humanity are an unanswered question.[1]

C. S. Lewis wrote a book entitled *The Problem of Pain*, which answers some of the questions suffering raises. But when suffering touched him personally in the death of his wife to cancer, he wrote a quite different book entitled *A Grief Observed*. Instead of answering questions, this time he was asking them: "Go to Him when your need is desperate, when all other help is vain, and what do you find? A door slammed in your face, and a sound of bolting and double bolting on the inside. After that, silence. You may as well turn away. The longer you wait, the more emphatic the silence will become. There are no lights in the windows. It might be an empty house. Was it ever inhabited? It seemed so once. And that seeming was as strong as this. What can this mean? Why is He so present a commander in our time of prosperity and so very absent a help in time of trouble?"

As Lewis trudged through his grief, his steps gradually grew lighter. Only then did he find the strength to reflect upon God's silence: "I have gradually been coming to feel that the door is no longer shut and bolted. Was it my own frantic need that slammed it in my face? The time when there is nothing at all in your soul except a cry for help may be just the time when God can't give it: you are like the drowning man who can't be helped because he clutches and grabs. Perhaps your own reiterated cries deafen you to the voice you hoped to hear."

The longer Lewis walked down the darkened corridors of his own grief, the closer he got to a window which shed light on his unanswered questions: "When I lay these questions before God I get no answer. But a rather special sort of 'No answer.' It is not the locked door. It is more like a silent, certainly not uncompassionate, gaze. As though He shook His head not in refusal but waiving the question. Like, 'Peace, child; you don't understand.'"[2]

I have learned with Lewis that God's silence to my questions is not a door slammed in my face. But for now and for the foreseeable future, I may not receive the answers I came to find.

– 22 –

The Missing Pieces in Suffering

ONE THING I always liked about baseball was that there was nothing ambiguous about the game. You looked up at the scoreboard and you knew exactly how many runs your team had, how many outs, and how many innings were left to play. Nothing ambiguous about that.

If it was a tie game after nine innings, you played extra innings until someone scored a run. One team went home the winner. The other team went home the loser. Nothing ambiguous about that.

There were boundaries chalked down the first and third baselines. If you hit a ball within the lines, it was fair. If you hit it outside the lines, it was foul.

Nothing ambiguous about that. And, if there ever was, an umpire stood ready to clear it up.

If only life could be like baseball.

If only we could look up and find out what the score was in our suffering, see how we were doing and how many innings we had left before it was all over. If only there were boundaries that made some types of suffering out-of-bounds. If only there was an umpire to jump in and settle the disputes.

149

It's not difficult to understand why some people look at life's ambiguities and conclude that the game isn't being played fairly. That's what this man concluded, who wrote to comment on my comeback from cancer:

> Dear Dave,
>
> I'm happy that you beat cancer, but according to the news release I'm hearing, you said, "It was a miracle from God." I have a problem with that. Do you think the people on Flight 232 that crashed in Iowa and died were hoping for a miracle? What about the 30 million people who died in World War II? Do you think they might have asked for divine help? Or the 6 million Jews that died in the ovens? Why didn't God give them the miracle they asked for?

Those are good questions, questions I sometimes ask myself. But in doing so, I am careful not to confuse life with God. Life is unfair, sometimes brutally so; God isn't.

But that begs the question: Why doesn't God intervene to make life more fair, to make his "will be done on earth as it is in heaven"? Especially why doesn't he intervene on behalf of one of his own children? I'm thinking of Laura. This letter from one of Laura's friends tells us her story:

> Dear Dave,
>
> This summer I questioned God for the first time in my life. I worked at a summer camp with 95% Jewish children. After my first week there I got involved in a Bible study with three other Christian counselors. Things were going really well until July 27, 1991. Half of us counselors had the day off. Most of us went to the beach, but a few went their own separate ways, including Laura. Laura was a girl in our Bible study. That day she took a hike by herself. She

never returned. The police found her body the next day. She had been raped by more than one person, and both her arms and legs were broken. I know Laura is in heaven, but her death affected me like nothing ever had in my entire life. I have questioned the violence of her death and my faith in God.

My heart broke when I read that letter. It caused me to question God, too. The young woman who wrote the letter told me in the postscript that Proverbs 3:5–6 were Laura's favorite verses. It stuck in my mind because it's one of my favorite passages, too: "Trust in the Lord with all your heart and lean not on your own understanding; in all your ways acknowledge him, and he will make your paths straight."

Where was God when Laura took that path through the woods? Why didn't he come to the aid of someone who trusted him the way she did?

I don't know where he was. I don't understand why he didn't come.

Life is a puzzle where many of the pieces don't fit. Especially at first, when the puzzle is dumped in our lap. It takes a while to sort through the pieces, to turn them all right side up, to see the overall pattern, to spot the connections. I don't think God holds it against us when we can't understand everything that happens in this jigsaw world of ours. Especially at first. And especially because some of the key pieces to that puzzle are missing.

In the first two chapters of the book of Job, we find a missing piece to the puzzle of Job's suffering. And finding it, we understand something of the "why" of his suffering. Job was never given that piece. At the end of the book he was given an audience with God, but not the piece that would have made sense of his suffering.

Why?

Maybe it was because God wanted Job to trust him. If that's the reason, could he want any less from us? Maybe what he wants is for us to put together as much of life's puzzle as we can, and then to trust him with the missing pieces—however many those pieces may be, however large, however gaping the holes that are left in our theology as a result.

The question then changes from being "Why, God?" to "Can I trust him with my unanswered questions?"

In the book *The Hiding Place*, Corrie ten Boom learned to trust her father with her unanswered questions. She had overheard a discussion about sexual immorality, and she didn't understand one of the words the adults used. Later she asked her father about it. He realized whatever answer he gave would be beyond the reach of a little girl who didn't know what sex was, let alone the misuse of sex:

> He turned to look at me, as he always did when answering a question, but to my surprise he said nothing. At last he stood up, lifted his traveling case from the rack over our heads, and set it on the floor.
>
> "Will you carry it off the train, Corrie?" he said.
>
> I stood up and tugged at it. It was crammed with the watches and spare parts he had purchased that morning.
>
> "It's too heavy," I said.
>
> "Yes," he said. "And it would be a pretty poor father who would ask his little girl to carry such a load. It's the same way, Corrie, with knowledge. Some knowledge is too heavy for children. When you are older and stronger you can bear it. For now you must trust me to carry it for you."

And I was satisfied. More than satisfied—wonderfully at peace. There were answers to this and all my hard questions—for now I was content to leave them in my father's keeping.[1]

Maybe the answers are, at least for now, too difficult to bear. Jesus said, "Blessed are those who mourn" not because he promised their questions would be answered but because he promised their hearts would be comforted.

When our hearts are broken and our eyes are blinded with tears, maybe we don't need answers nearly as much as we need a father's lap to crawl onto and his shoulder where we can bury our face and cry.

– 23 –

Dave Dravecky Day

On OCTOBER 5, 1991, the Giants invited me back to San Francisco for a special celebration in my honor: "Dave Dravecky Day." I'm not one for a whole lot of attention, but I thought it was wonderful what the Giants wanted to do. I was excited about seeing old friends and coming back one more time to Candlestick Park.

Jan and I arrived at the stadium early Saturday morning for a press conference. There were a lot of new faces with the Giants. A lot of old faces had moved on, like the changing of the guard. Atlee Hammaker had been released and signed with the Padres. Brett Butler had signed as a free agent with the Dodgers. Will Clark and Scott Garrelts were a couple of former teammates who were still there.

Not only had the ballclub changed; I had changed. I looked at baseball in a totally different way now. Now I was someone on the outside looking in. I was no longer a ballplayer; I was just a fan. These guys were no longer my teammates; they were just my friends.

My whole family came to San Francisco for this special tribute. My parents were there along with my brothers and their wives. My brothers liked the fact that I was a big-league ballplayer, but they never made a big deal out of it. I always appreciated that about them. Having them around me that day made me appreciate my roots and the history we had shared together as a family.

The Giants were playing the Dodgers that day. It was a must game for Los Angeles. If they lost this one, they wouldn't be going to the playoffs.

The rivalry between the two teams was an intense one. Playing against the Dodgers always brought out the best in me; I once pitched a one-hitter against them. Everyone on our team played their best against the Dodgers. You had to if you wanted to beat them.

It was great being in the clubhouse again, the slightly pungent smell of glove leather lingering in the air like pipe tobacco. Man, I loved that smell.

The Giants provided me with a uniform. Putting it on brought back a lot of fond memories. But it took a while to put it on, partly because of my arm and partly because of the weight I had gained. Scott Garrelts, who was recovering from reconstructive surgery in his right elbow, helped squeeze me into it.

Once I was suited up, I left the clubhouse and looked out across the stadium. The finely manicured grass was almost an iridescent green. The bright orange seats were starting to fill. The U.S. and California flags rippled in the breeze. And arching over it all was a big blue dome of sky.

I was caught up in the wonder of it all, of just being alive and being there in that ballpark. I felt like a seven-year-old kid, seeing it all for the first time. "Take me out to the ballgame. Take me out to the crowd. Buy me some peanuts and Cracker Jack. I don't care if I ever get back."

Dave Dravecky Day

Theme music from the Olympics boomed over the public-address system, and a throng of children and adults burst from the center field gates. The people in the stands stood and clapped as they spread over the field. High over their heads they carried banners and placards. I was overwhelmed with the sentiments they expressed:

DAVE, ALWAYS A GIANT
DRAVECKY #43
YOU ARE A GIANT HERO
THANKS FOR THE HOPE
GOOD LUCK, DAVE!
GOD BLESS U.
THANKS FOR THE MEMORIES

The announcer's voice pierced through the collective hush of that shirtsleeved Saturday afternoon: "Faith, fortitude, and fearless determination in the face of adversity. Courage is Dave Dravecky."

As his words echoed through the stands, the fans clapped again. I walked to the platform that had been set up on the pitcher's mound, my teammates following behind me. They sat on the grass as Hank Greenwald stepped up to the microphone. His words were addressed to me: "Many would gladly give their arms to see you out there again." What touched me so much was that I knew what he said was true.

During the ceremony the Giants gave out the "Courageous Kid Award" to five kids who faced cancer with uncommon courage: Andrew Slade from Fremont, Ryan Dzygunik from San Mateo, Katie Brown from Fairfield, Cameron Bradley from Hollister, and Mollie Back from San Jose. I was taken with the courage of these young kids. In a lot of ways they were going through struggles much greater than mine, because they had to face adversity at such an early age.

I stepped up to the microphone and addressed the crowd: "God has allowed me to be a vehicle to help young kids like these. They are the real heroes, the five kids behind me. I wish I could be on this mound today, but I can't. I want you to know, though, that putting on a Giants' uniform meant more to me than anything in my professional career."

A message flashed across the giant screen high in the stands: WE LOVE YOU, DAVE.

When I saw it, a rush of memories came at me all at once, memories of when the words WELCOME BACK, DAVE were flashed across that same screen during my comeback game. I wouldn't be coming back, but I would be taking their love with me.

When the ceremonies concluded, one of the boys, who had had a forequarter amputation just like mine, was standing beside me. I looked at him and said: "Let's do a stub shake." I bent down, and we did a phantom handshake by rubbing our nubs together. We smiled at each other without saying anything. We didn't have to. There was a bond between us that went beyond words.

A convertible drove Jan and I around the perimeter of the ballpark as a nostalgic duet between Natalie Cole and her father, the great Nat King Cole, filled the stadium with the song "Unforgettable." I would remember baseball the way Natalie Cole remembered her father. With warmth and affection. With love and gratitude. With memories that would always be . . . unforgettable.

As we drove by the stands, a wave of applause followed us around the field.

I lifted my cap to the crowd.

Dave Dravecky Day

It was my last hurrah. I felt a sense of closure as we circled the ballpark, a closing of the final chapter of my career as a professional athlete.

I came to Candlestick Park to say thank you. And to say good-bye. Thank you to the Giants and the fans. Good-bye to a game I loved.

Just a few minutes ago I had been standing on the platform on the pitcher's mound, daydreaming, thinking how great it would be to be able to go to the dugout, get my glove, and pitch against the Dodgers.

But it was just a daydream. I could never come back. I knew that.

Tragedy pushes us through a one-way door, and once we pass through it, we can never return to the way life was before that tragedy. A parent who loses a daughter to leukemia can never again go back to her bedroom and kiss that little girl goodnight, or read her bedtime stories, or kneel beside her bed and pray. A Vietnam vet with his legs blown off can never go back to the sidewalks of his youth where he skipped so kiddishly and carefree. A woman who has been brutally raped can never go back to a time of innocence when, as a starry-eyed little girl, she dreamed of being swept off her feet by some handsome prince.

We can't go back, no matter how much we ache to do so. All we can do is give thanks for what once was, for the good that was there, for the happy times that were had, for the laughter, for the love, for the memories that were shared. Then, saying good-bye to those times and to those loved ones, we can put our hand in the hand of him who gave orbit to the sun and the moon and the stars, and trust that he has a course for our lives as well.

– 24 –

Dealing with Depression

DURING THAT WEEKEND in San Francisco I started experiencing stomach problems. Actually they started two weeks before, but now they were getting worse. By the time we returned to Ohio, I was having all sorts of abdominal pain. One day the pain would be a burning sensation on the right side of my stomach. The next day it would be on the left. Other times it felt as though a knife were stabbing me. And then at night I would sometimes wake up with my esophagus burning like crazy. The more this happened, the more I worried.

I worried not so much about the intensity of the pain but about its origin. Had the cancer returned? Had it spread throughout my body, wrapping itself around my internal organs? Was that what I was feeling?

Up to this point I felt I had everything together. "I can handle this," I would say to myself anytime a new obstacle came my way. But this time I wasn't so sure. Prior to these unexplained pains, death seemed remote, probably because I had suppressed the idea. But now for the first time in my life, I thought about it. I thought about it a lot. I remember in the past telling talk show hosts how I wasn't afraid of dying. Death seemed so remote then, but now that I could hear its footsteps, I was scared.

I had always avoided the question "What scares me?" because I felt that Christians weren't supposed to be afraid. "Fear not," the Bible says. "Let not your heart be troubled" . . . "Be anxious for nothing" . . . "Perfect love casts out fear." And yet fear and worry were eating my lunch.

Then I started getting cluster headaches. The pain was excruciating. One time the pain got so bad that I wrapped my head in a pillow and banged it against the wall to try to get some relief. My phantom pains were also intensifying.

In the wake of the physical pain came the mental anguish. I started remembering faces of people I had met in the hospital who had died. The faces haunted me, but I kept brushing them aside. I had to keep going, I told myself. I couldn't stop to think about these things. There wasn't time in my schedule. I had to keep going.

I kept going for the rest of the month, jetting around the country, speaking in Pittsburgh, Reno, Decatur, Slippery Rock, Sioux Falls.

"WHEN DAVE ARRIVED home, I could tell he was beat, not just physically but emotionally as well. He was short with the kids, and then he yelled at me. I went in the backyard and stood against a tree and cried. When I finally dried my eyes and came inside, Dave was sitting on the bed.

"'You're better off without me,' he said. It was a cry for comfort, a way to express his hurt without asking for help.

"'Why do you say that?'

"'Do you know the hell it is to live with one arm?'

162

"I could tell he wanted to cry, but he couldn't. So I sat down beside him, holding him in my arms, and I cried for him."

JAN'S COMFORT HELPED, at least for the moment.

The last weekend in October I was in Dallas, speaking four times on Sunday morning and working on a documentary film project all that afternoon.

When I was there, I couldn't wait to get home and be with Jan and the kids. The feeling bordered on desperation. It was as if I were drifting downriver, approaching a deadly waterfall, and I was swimming against swift currents, groping to catch an overhanging limb or grab onto a boulder to stop me from being swept away. I was only thirty-five. I was too young to die. I had too much to live for. My kids needed me. Jan needed me.

From Dallas I flew to northern California, where I spoke eight times in five days, making stops at San Jose, Sacramento, Modesto, and Merced. I spoke to over ten thousand people during those five days. It was an exhausting experience. By the end of that time I was hanging on by a thread. When I arrived home for the weekend, the thread broke, and I crashed. I was shaking, constipated, nauseated, and had all sorts of strange internal pains. I walked around the house like a zombie, totally exhausted.

I woke up the next morning, lying in bed, feeling depressed. Fortunately Jan wasn't spooning out the same medicine I had given her when she was depressed. She wasn't telling me to snap out of it or get with it. She understood. She had been there and back.

When You Can't Come Back

"I HAD KNOWN for some time now that Dave was suffering from burnout. Dr. Townsend said it, and I saw it firsthand. The medication Dave was taking for his phantom pains put him in a terrible mood, but I didn't know how bad he felt until one day when he came to me and admitted it.

"'I'm afraid,' he said. 'I don't feel good.'

"'Dave, you probably have an ulcer.'

"'No. I'm afraid I have a tumor.'

"'You know what's wrong? You're depressed.'

"'You're probably right.'

"I couldn't believe my ears. Dave actually agreed with me. And he didn't even put up a fight. We compared symptoms, and it was amazing how his paralleled mine. Then he really threw me for a loop.

"'I'm so sorry for everything, Jan. I never knew this is how you felt. Boy, I feel like a heel for making fun of you, for not taking you to get help. I'm so sorry.'

"I don't know how many times Dave said he was sorry, but it was a lot. I told him it was all right and that I understood."

BUT NO AMOUNT of understanding, even from Jan, could pull me out of the valley I was in. Suddenly all the feelings I had buried for so long began coming to the surface. I was sick of not being able to fit into my clothes because of all the weight I had gained. I was sick of being an amputee, having my wife cut my meat, tie my tie, tuck in my shirttail. And I was sick of being a hypocrite. I was on the road giving people the impression I had it all together, when here I was at home with the wheels falling off my life.

Dealing with Depression

"I HATED SEEING Dave like this, not only because of all the pain he was in, but because it reminded me of all the pain I had been in when I had gone through my depression.

"I decided to let him sleep in and to let him do all the fun things he enjoyed doing, like going with Bob to his construction sites and talking with the workers there. I made sure the work in his study was done so he wouldn't have to be bothered by that. I put restrictions on what he could and couldn't do when he was out speaking—no autographs, no extra meetings. I made him promise that all he would do was to go and speak and then come home. I even let him watch all the TV he wanted, without complaining."

As I SAT ON the couch, flipping through the channels on the remote, I thought about the past two years of my life. I regretted wasting so much time. How many hours had I parked myself in front of this tube, flipping through the channels, hoping for an old John Wayne movie, a heated debate on CNN's "Crossfire," or some sporting event? I had given that television countless hours of my life. What had it given me in return?

I pressed the off button and sprawled out on the cushions. I began to tune in to thoughts about my faith and about my family.

Saint Paul said that for him to live was Christ and to die was gain. I wanted to feel that way, but I didn't. Death was not a gain to me. It was a loss of everything I held close to my heart. I didn't want to die. I didn't want to leave. I wanted to be here to watch Jonathan grow up and play sports, to walk Tiffany down the aisle on her wedding day. And I wanted to be here to live with Jan. I thought about her remarrying, having another man take my place, a man who would make her laugh, who would raise our kids, who would sleep in my bed. The thought was more than I could bear. I wanted to grow old with Jan, not die young with cancer.

I questioned whether I had the strength to fight this one last battle. I questioned whether I even had the will to fight.

I finally went to see Dr. McGowen, and he gave me a complete checkup. Over the past year I had taken all kinds of antibiotics, pain medication, and anti-inflammatory medication. Often I had taken these on an empty stomach, and that stomach was shouting, "Enough already!" The doctor said I had a peptic ulcer, probably brought on by all the medication I had been taking and by all the stress I had been under. I confided in him about my fear of the cancer's spreading, about my fear of dying, and about being depressed.

Opening up to Dr. McGowen really helped. He didn't condemn me or lecture me. He told me I was starting to face reality about the loss of my arm, and that was the first constructive step I had taken in the grieving process.

It was normal to grieve, he told me, not a lack of faith. It was normal to feel fearful when unexplained pain shoots through your body. It was normal for my stomach to be reacting to the stress I was under and to all the medication. It was my body telling me to slow down, to relax, to stop suppressing my feelings. One by one, Dr. McGowen addressed the problems I was having.

To alleviate my fears or to confirm them, Dr. McGowen had a CAT scan done on my abdomen. It came out negative. There was no trace of cancer. But even that good news didn't change how low I felt.

Dealing with Depression

The next morning I dragged myself out of bed and took a shower. After I toweled off and put on my pants, I looked in the bathroom mirror. Staring back at me was this dumpy, disfigured man who couldn't even cut his own meat. *How disgusting*, I thought. But that's as far as I let the feeling get out. I turned my eyes from the man in the mirror and just continued dressing. When Jan came in, the feeling resurfaced.

"How can you love me like this?" I asked.

"I'd love you if you didn't have *any* arms," she said.

I wanted to cry, but I couldn't. A good, hard cry would have done me a lot of good, but I just couldn't do it.

I've always had a difficult time expressing my feelings. But it goes deeper than that. I've always had a hard time having feelings at all. And sometimes I think I'm numb to the feelings of others. I remember when I was a kid, a friend of mine took a bad fall on his bike and was really hurt. All I did was laugh. Here the guy was all banged up, and I couldn't feel anything for him. I couldn't enter into his pain. It was all just so much slapstick comedy to me.

In 1970, when my grandfather died, I didn't cry. We were very close, and his death hurt, but I held it in. I don't know why. My parents both cried, but I didn't.

Tapping into those feelings has been like chipping away at a frozen river to get it flowing again. My life has been so rushed the past couple of years, I haven't had time to think about everything that's happened to me. I haven't had time to feel. Maybe with my life slowing down a little now, some of those feelings will begin to thaw.

I've seen some evidences of it already. One day while I was driving the car and listening to a song, I started crying. For no reason, I just started crying. Another time I was speaking at a church, and during the song service, tears started to roll down my face. Something was stirring inside me, some spring-like sensation that was beginning to melt my heart.

I finally opened up to Jan and let my feelings out. I told her of my fears about cancer, about dying, about her marrying someone else. It was hard for me to do, but after I did, it felt as if a huge weight was lifted from my shoulders.

I told her, too, how much I was struggling with being dependent on someone else. Before, when I was a pitcher, I called the signals. *I* threw the ball; nobody did it for me. I put it where *I* wanted it. In spite of my retirement from baseball, in spite of the loss of my arm, there was still a self-sufficient athlete inside me that didn't want to come to terms with the fact that he needed help.

Monday I spoke in Youngstown, Ohio, then flew to West Palm Beach in Florida to speak to "A Gathering of Men" meeting. Tuesday night, November 12, 1991, I shared with them something of my comeback story, of the subsequent surgeries, and of my relationship with Christ. But I didn't go into a lot of detail as I usually would've done. Instead I decided to let down my defenses and let them into my life. I let them know what was going on now, not what went on three years ago. I shared with them how overwhelmed I was by the number of speaking requests that had come in for the next year—over seven hundred. I told them that I was so busy I didn't have time for God, my wife, or my kids.

"Here I am standing before you," I told them, "sharing the importance of these three things in my life, and I'm not practicing what I'm preaching. Here I am telling you men how important your commitment to your family is, and my family has hardly seen me the past two weeks. And when they did, I was so worn out I had nothing left to give them. What does that say about *me*, about *my* priorities?"

I told them about the physical problems I was experiencing, and about the depression. I told them that I thought God was trying to teach me an important lesson. God desired fellowship with me, but if I wanted it, I was going to have to slow down and reevaluate the direction my life was heading.

The response of the men was incredible. They came up afterward and thanked me, many of them telling me how they were battling against depression, too, and how they had been guilty of putting their jobs first.

When I got back to my hotel room, I felt this tremendous sense of relief. I felt set free from the public perception of who Dave Dravecky was. He wasn't this able-to-leap-tall-buildings-in-a-single-bound Super-Christian. He was human. He had doubts and fears and hurts in his life, just like anybody else.

The relief I felt that night was only a temporary reprieve.

Shortly after I arrived home from my speaking engagement in West Palm Beach, I received a letter in the mail with an article on depression. I appreciated the letter. It was kind and gracious. But the article wasn't any help. It claimed to be the biblical answer to depression. It quoted a few verses and then gave this advice: "Force your mind into sunshine thoughts. Do this especially when your mind starts the 'instant replays' of old fears and depressive thoughts."

I'm sorry, but to me, forcing your mind into "sunshine thoughts" when you're going through a time of depression is like standing in the rain and denying there's a storm. Faith is not denying the weather that sweeps over your life. It's believing that behind the clouds and beyond the storms waits a faithful God.

At the moment, though, I couldn't see him. The cloud that hung over me was too thick. It was the impenetrable darkness of that cloud that caused me to do something I've never done before. I called Atlee Hammaker and asked if he would go with me on November 15 to Memphis, where I was supposed to speak at a financial convention for the Morgan-Keagan Company.

"I need you, Atlee. I need your fellowship, your encouragement. I'm really down."

I couldn't believe the words coming out of my mouth. I actually reached out to someone and asked for help.

Atlee and I spent two-and-a-half days in Memphis. It was great. He's such an understanding friend. We've been through so much together. He knew me when I was just a no-name ballplayer, struggling to secure a place in the Giants' lineup. We roomed together a lot when the team was on the road. He knows how lonely and demanding that kind of life is. He knows the pain of surgery, having had both his shoulder and his knee operated on. He knows the pressure a big-league pitcher lives with.

Most of all, he knows me.

Best of all, he accepts me just the way I am.

When we are together, we're always at ease. We have so much shared history, so many things in common, that we're never worried about what the other person is thinking or whether we've said the wrong thing or anything like that.

During that time in Memphis we talked about some of what I was going through, how difficult the speaking schedule had been, the struggles Jan and I were experiencing, about life after baseball. I didn't open up a lot; it was just being with an old friend who understood . . . that's what meant so much to me.

Later that month our families got together for the Thanksgiving holidays. I told him not to plan anything, that I just wanted to be there with him. I had sunk even lower by then, and that week I never needed a friend more than I needed Atlee.

He shared with me about his depression. Then I opened up and shared about mine. I shared about the mental turmoil and the stress and the fear of dying.

Neither one of us shared anything very profound or life-changing. Nothing really important happened. And yet it was all so important.

– 25 –

Where We Are Now

THE MEDICATION for my ulcer helped my stomach to heal, and the unexplained abdominal pains I had been so worried about began to go away. The break in my traveling schedule gave me the rest I so desperately needed. I started getting my strength back, and I hired a trainer to put me on a regular exercise routine. As my physical health improved, so did my emotional health. Slowly with the help of counseling from Dr. Sommers, the cloud I had been under lifted.

Now instead of denying the losses in my life, I'm learning to grieve over them. Instead of holding my feelings in, I'm learning to express them. Instead of throwing phones against the wall, I'm learning to listen to the person on the other end of the line.

After my bout with depression ended, I prayed, "Thank you, God, for the wake-up call." I am so much more awake now, alert not only to eternity but to the gift of life here on earth. Funny how a brush with death, even an imagined brush, makes you more appreciative of life. I am more aware of how precious each day is; how sacred a moment is; how it, too, is a gift, something that comes to us by grace, something that is to be held carefully and treasured.

So many people, it seems, let those sacred moments slip by without notice because they are preoccupied with the future, with their hopes and dreams and plans. We can be so intent on looking down the road at what we want out of life that we miss the beautiful scenery along the way. Playing catch in the backyard with your son. Reading to your daughter nestled next to you on the couch. Feeding the ducks on a walk around the pond with your wife.

The beautiful scenery along the way. It goes past our window in a blur as we push the speed limit to arrive at our destination. No thank you. I've been down that road before. And I've seen the wreckage.

I've seen ballplayers lose everything meaningful in life on the road to what they thought would give them meaning and purpose and happiness. I've seen them lose their marriage, their family, their own soul, en route to getting the big bucks contract, the fancy car, the beautiful home. No, I'll plan for the future, but you won't catch me living there. There's too much treasure in a day. And I don't want any of it slipping between my fingers.

Having groped in the darkness of a depression, I feel more sensitive to the people around me. The depression I experienced was just a taste of what Jan had gone through. I feel bad for letting her suffer so long without getting her the help she needed, but at least now I feel *something*. Before, I couldn't relate at all to what she was going through. Now I'm beginning to understand. Now I'm beginning to learn something about emotions. I stress the word "beginning." I still have a long way to go.

Where We Are Now

I wish I were further along with regard to relationships, but I'm not. Here I am, a thirty-five-year-old man; I've been a Christian for eleven years, and yet I'm only three months old in learning how to express my needs and to receive love from other people.

But I'm growing in that area. By the time this book is published and in the bookstores, I'll be a year old! And next year, I'll be two years old. Hopefully each year I'll grow and mature in that area of my life.

I'm growing in other areas of my life, too. I feel more appreciative for Jan. I love her now more than I ever have before. I am thankful for having a second chance at life, to be able to watch Jonathan and Tiffany grow up, to be able to grow old with my high school sweetheart.

Jan and I are just now stepping out of the wilderness. We're beginning to feel a little cool grass under our feet instead of the hot sand we've been used to for the past two years. It's a good feeling.

Looking back, we have learned that the wilderness is part of the landscape of faith, and every bit as essential as the mountaintop. On the mountaintop we are overwhelmed by God's presence. In the wilderness we are overwhelmed by his absence. Both places should bring us to our knees; the one, in utter awe; the other, in utter dependence.

One by one the wilderness took from us everything we had depended upon in place of God. It took away our physical health, our mental and emotional health, our church, our friends, and even took us away from each other. All those things that we relied on for our source of strength were gone. We were forced to turn to God because there was nowhere else to turn. But at times in the wilderness he seemed to be distant, if not absent altogether.

But just when our mouths were parched and Jan and I felt we would die of thirst, he provided a well in the wilderness—Dr. McGowen. Just when we were completely disoriented, he provided a sign pointing the way—Dr. Townsend. Just when it looked as if every trace of him had vanished, he provided a flower—Sealy Yates. Just when it felt as if I were going to die from sunstroke, he provided shade—Atlee Hammaker.

Through them we learned that God was not absent in the wilderness. He was there. We saw him. In the caring eyes of a family doctor. In the sympathetic voice of a psychologist. In the helping hands of a friend. In the comfortable presence of a fellow ballplayer.

As Jan and I reflect on our time in the wilderness, we learned a lot. We learned to walk by faith rather than by sight. Where did Job say, "Though he slay me, yet will I trust him"? In the wilderness of his own suffering. Where did David say, "O God, My God! How I search for you! How I thirst for you in a parched and weary land where there is no water"? In the wilderness when he hid from his enemies. Where did Jesus say, "Man does not live by bread alone but by every word that proceeds from the mouth of God"? In the wilderness when he fought off the temptations of the devil.

It was in the wilderness, too, that Jan and I learned to trust God, even though at times every visible trace of him had vanished. The spiritual starkness of the wilderness was what was so difficult to deal with. But we finally came to the point that Habakkuk did when he prayed: "Though the fig tree does not bud and there are no grapes on the vines, though the olive crop fails and the fields produce no food, though there are no sheep in the pen and no cattle in the stalls, yet I will rejoice in the Lord, I will be joyful to God my Savior. The Sovereign Lord is my strength; he makes my feet like the feet of a deer, and he enables me to go on the heights"(Hab. 3:17–19).

Jan and I can't say we had the feet of a deer as we went through the wilderness. Ours were a lot more clumsy than that. But I can honestly say we had the will to walk. In our heart of hearts we wanted to please God, to trust him, to love him, to obey him.

And I truly believe he was pleased.

Even with our stumbles.

– 26 –

Finding the Grace

IN 1968, FIFTY PERCENT of the people with my type of cancer had to undergo amputation. Today, that number has dropped to three or four percent, thanks to such excellent research centers as Sloan-Kettering, and thanks to such outstanding doctors as Dr. Brennan.

But to talk with Dr. Brennan you would get a different picture: "Amputation is a failure for the doctor, and on top of that you feel this great sense of sadness for cutting away a part of the patient's life. A generation from now, doctors will look back on this type of procedure and say I was a barbarian."

I think Dr. Brennan was being too hard on himself when he told me that. I certainly didn't feel that way. Better my limb than my life. But if in a generation from now doctors look back and call him a barbarian, they will only be able to do so because of the pioneering work he and other dedicated doctors have done. Dr. Brennan had done everything within his power. I didn't expect any more. After all, he was a doctor, not a miracle worker.

I spent only six days in the hospital, and then I went home. It was there that I experienced some pretty severe "phantom pains." Even though my arm was gone, I could still feel pain in the place where my arm used to be. It was weird. I mean, we're talking *Twilight Zone* weird. I'd get this burning sensation in my fingertips—only I had no fingertips! But I did have the pain. That was real. Sometimes the pain got so intense it was distracting. To manage this pain I had been given a powerful narcotic when I left the hospital. But I was concerned because it was addictive. I went to Dr. McGowen to see if he could give me something else. He prescribed a drug commonly used to treat neuropathic pain, the type of pain people have when they get shingles. Even though the nerves in my arm had been severed, the nerve pathways from my brain, down my spinal cord, and leading to that area toward my arm were all still functioning. The drug I was prescribed dulled the memory of these pathways and in time gave me a measure of relief.

Three weeks later I went to Orlando, Florida, for the Christian Booksellers Convention, where I was interviewed by a woman from *Good Morning, America*. During the interview I was struggling with some of those phantom pains. It felt as if someone had taken a fork and jabbed it into my hand. The last thing I felt like doing was giving an interview. But when I saw the segment on television, I was glad I had gone through with it. I was particularly touched by how Charlie Gibson introduced the segment.

"Facing cancer takes courage," he said; "it takes determination. Still, most people who survive and cope with the disease can eventually return to their jobs and get back to work. The case of Dave Dravecky, followed by millions of people, is unique. Once a fine, left-handed pitcher in the major leagues for San Francisco, last month his cancer-riddled arm was amputated. Where does someone find the grace to cope with a tragic irony like that?"

Finding the Grace

If you are an English teacher, your ear might have caught the dangling modifier. But what caught my ear was the word "grace."

It's one of the most beautiful words in the whole world. Grace is a gift. The smell of hot roasted peanuts at the ballpark is grace. The passing cloud that shades you in the center field bleachers is grace. The ability Babe Ruth had to hit home runs came to him by grace. It was due to the fact that he had the best hand-eye coordination of probably anyone in baseball history. He worked to develop his ability, but he did nothing to deserve it. It was a gift.

So then where does someone find grace, especially the grace to face tragedy?

In the hands of a heavenly Father. He gives us the grace to face life's uncertainties, its disappointments, and its tragedies.

There's a story in *The Hiding Place* where the young Corrie ten Boom sees a baby who has died and curiously touches its face. The feel of the cold and lifeless skin startles her. Suddenly she realizes that if death could take this little baby, no one was safe, not even the loved ones in her family. The thought terrified her and caused her to burst into tears. Listen how Corrie's father helps her understand the grace of God:

> Father sat down on the edge of the narrow bed. "Corrie," he began gently, "when you and I go to Amsterdam— when do I give you your ticket?"
>
> [She] sniffed a few times, considering this.
>
> "Why, just before we get on the train."
>
> "Exactly. And our wise Father in heaven knows when we're going to need things, too. Don't run out ahead of Him, Corrie. When the time comes that some of us will

have to die, you will look into your heart and find the strength you need—just in time."[1]

I'm not getting through the loss of my arm because I am a great coper. I'm getting through it because I have a Father in heaven who is a great giver. *He* is where I find the grace. At the time I need strength, he puts it in my heart or provides it through someone who is close to me, whether that's a family doctor or simply a friend. I don't earn it. I don't deserve it. I don't bring it about. It's a gift. And that is how I am able to cope with the "tragic irony" of losing my arm.

– 27 –

A Father's Ache

WHEN MY FAMILY was in San Francisco for "Dave Dravecky Day," something happened that I'd like to share with you. It was one of those small things that sometimes happens in a family, one of those small, sweet things you savor the rest of your life.

The day after the ballgame the whole family went to Sausalito. We got to spend some quality time together there, something we hadn't been able to do for a long time, and I felt closer to them than I ever had. I think they felt that way, too.

Later that day a friend of mine invited us all over for barbecue. Jan and I had to leave early, so after we ate, we said our good-byes and left. Just before we started the car, my dad caught up with us. He leaned his head into the window and kissed me on the cheek.

"I love you," he said.

I looked into his eyes and smiled. "I love you, too."

It was the only time in the past few years we had been able to express feelings like that to each other.

Dad's eyes filled with tears. "It means so much to me having all the family together like this."

It brought to the surface the ache in my heart for my father's love.

"HEY, DAD, you wanna play catch?"

How many times had I asked him that when I was a kid? I can't even begin to count.

You won't be surprised, then, that I cry when I hear that same question asked in the closing scene of the movie *Field of Dreams*. For those of you unfamiliar with the film, it's kind of a Frank Capra, feel-good type of movie, a baseball-story equivalent to *It's a Wonderful Life*.

Only it's not a story about baseball.

It's a story about a relationship between a son and his father. In his prime, John Kinsella had been a minor league ballplayer. But he couldn't make it in the minors and finally had to quit to support his family. He tried to teach the game to his son Ray, hoping the boy would catch his dream and one day make it as a professional ballplayer.

But by the time Ray was ten, playing baseball was like eating vegetables. He hated it. By the time he was fourteen, he rebelled. He put up his glove and refused to play catch anymore. When he was seventeen, he got in a fight with his father and left home for good. The father died sometime later, and the breach in their relationship was something Ray Kinsella had to learn to live with.

The author of the story uses an extended metaphor to illustrate the pain of that breached relationship. The image he uses is of eight White Sox players who were banned from baseball for conspiring to lose the 1919 World Series. The commissioner of baseball ruled that they not only couldn't play the sport anymore, they couldn't even so much as put on a professional baseball uniform.

The ache those eight men had for baseball was the same type of ache that son had for his father. Just as they couldn't put on a uniform and play baseball, so he couldn't put on his glove and play catch with his dad. Though he didn't realize it, Ray longed for his father's acceptance and approval. He longed for it the way those eight ballplayers longed to be accepted and approved by the sport they loved.

If only Ray could turn back the clock. If only he could take back those angry words. If only he could pick up that glove again and play catch with his dad.

The movies are one place where wishes like those are sometimes granted. And in this movie the son is granted his unspoken wish.

The story goes like this:

While Ray is walking in his Iowa cornfield, a strange voice whispers, "If you build it, he will come." For a fleeting moment he sees a glimpse of a ballfield. After racking his brain for the meaning of it all, he finally digs up part of his cornfield to build that ballfield. He waits and waits while his neighbors look on, thinking he's lost his mind.

But finally someone does come. Coming through the cornfield, through time, is Shoeless Joe Jackson, the most famous of the banned White Sox players. Eventually all eight of them are reunited on that magical field and get to play baseball once again.

Other cryptic messages come: "Ease his pain" . . . "Go the distance." And Ray is off on a quest to unravel them.

Other ballplayers come, too. The men invited a few other former players so they could have another team to play against.

After the game as the ballplayers are packing up, Shoeless Joe comes to Ray, smiling.

"What are you grinning at?" Ray asks.

Shoeless Joe points to the catcher and says to Ray, "If you build it, *he* will come."

Suddenly Ray recognizes the man. It's his father. Only it's a young, lean John Kinsella with the body he had during his prime. Ray also recognizes something else. The building of the field was not for Shoeless Joe. It was for Ray. The whole thing of making a ballfield had been so his father could come and "ease his pain"—Ray's pain—the pain he had as a result of the breach in their relationship.

Ray awkwardly tries to talk with him. After a few exchanges of congenial conversation, they say good-bye, and his father turns to go. But Ray has longed for this moment for years, and he won't let it slip away.

"Hey, Dad," he calls out with a crack in his voice. "You wanna play catch?"

His father turns and smiles. "I'd like that."

They toss the ball to each other, and the healing begins.

That final scene in the movie is a powerful image for the ache all of us have for our heavenly Father. We may not realize it, as Ray didn't, but it's there. We may resist our Father's dreams and rebel against his influence, but underneath it all we long for his embrace. We may run from him, the way Ray ran away from home, but we can't run away from the deepest longings of our heart—the longing to restore the breach in that relationship.

Jesus told a similar story in the parable of the prodigal son. It's called a parable because, like *Field of Dreams*, it is not a story just about one particular family. It is a story about us. All of us.

A Father's Ache

It's the story about a son who ran away from home. He wanted to be out from underneath his father's thumb, wanted to be in control of his life, make his own decisions, be his own boss. He wanted to live, really live, and to taste every fruit—however forbidden—that life had to offer.

But the fruit, sweet as it was at first, turned bitter. And he found himself in a distant country, without money and without food. He took a job tending the pigs of foreigners. Famished, he looked at the slop being fed the pigs and hungered for it. Then he came to his senses and realized that even his father's servants ate better than he did. That is when the prodigal son turned toward home.

On his way back the son worked out a confession. He had messed up his life so much; he wanted to do it right this time and make sure he didn't blow it. He rehearsed his speech again and again, making sure he got every word right.

When the son crested the last hill toward home, still a long way off, his father saw him. How many days had the father squinted at that horizon, searching for his son? How many sleepless nights had he sat up, hoping, praying, aching for his son's return?

When his son finally did return, the pent-up emotions burst from the father's heart. He ran as fast as he could, his heart overcome with joy, his eyes overflowing with tears. When he reached his son, there were no awkward pauses, no raised eyebrows, no stern looks. There were no lectures, no ridiculing remarks: "I *knew* when the money ran out, you'd come crawling back" . . . "Well, what have you got to say for yourself?" . . . "Look at you; you're a mess" . . . "You can come back, but only on one condition." There was no room in the father's heart for criticism because it was so filled with compassion. He threw his arms around his son's shoulders and showered him with kisses.

Awkwardly the son tried to frame the words to his confession, but the father heard none of it. Instead he hollered to his servants, "Quickly, bring the best robe and put it on him, put a ring on his hand and sandals on his feet! Kill the fattened calf and prepare a feast! Let's celebrate! For my son is alive! He's alive, and he's come home!"

God aches for the world the same way that father ached for his son.

I saw something of that ache in my own father's heart, as tears streamed down his face, as he kissed me, as he said: "I love you. It means so much to me having all the family together like this."

How far would a father go to demonstrate his love, to bring his family together?

– 28 –

Demonstration of a Father's Love

B<small>ABE</small> R<small>UTH</small> <small>IS</small> <small>TO</small> baseball what John 3:16 is to the Bible. If you know just one baseball player, it's probably the Babe. If you know just one Bible verse, it's probably John 3:16. "For God so loved the world that he gave his only begotten son, that whosoever would believe in him would not perish but have everlasting life."

God so ached for the return of this prodigal world that he gave up his only son to bring it home. I have to tell you honestly, I can't understand that. I can't fathom why he would do that. Jonathan is my only son, and there's no way I would give him up. Or Tiffany either. Not for anything. Not to get my arm back. Not to play baseball again. Not for the world.

And yet . . .

And yet that is why God gave his son—for the world. When his son entered that world, he was subjected to all its pain, all its misery, all its suffering.

He experienced the pain of being squeezed through a birth canal. He suffered the shame of innuendoes involving the legitimacy of his birth. He felt the pangs of hunger from his forty days in the wilderness. He knew the pain of rejection from his people, from his hometown, from his own family. He knew the sadness of having a friend die. He knew what it was like to be falsely accused. He knew the feeling of being hated simply because of his race.

He felt the refusal of heaven the night he anguished in prayer in the Garden of Gethsemane. He knew what it was like to be deserted by his closest friends, to be denied, to be betrayed. He knew the fists of Roman soldiers and the rods they slapped across his back. He knew what it was like to be mocked, as a crown of thorns was mashed into his head, a purple cape draped over his shoulders, and a reed placed in his hand. "Hail, King of the Jews." He knew the bite of the whip that tore away his flesh. He knew the fever that inflamed his open wounds. He knew the sharp iron of heavy spikes as they were pounded into his hands and feet. He felt the sting of insults thrust at him from the crowd. He knew the thirst of fever and dehydration as he hung on that rough-cut cross.

He knew the disorienting kind of suffering that prompts the question, "My God, my God, *why* have you forsaken me?" And he knew what it was like not to have a question like that answered.

"He was a man of sorrows, acquainted with grief."

While Jesus suffered on the cross, he had every reason to question God's love and to doubt his care. But when he approached death's door, he trusted his father to lead him across the threshold. "Father, into your hands I commit my spirit."

However unfair we may think God is in allowing a world where suffering exists, we have to give him credit for one thing. He played by his own rules. And he didn't play favorites.

"Although he was a son, he learned obedience from what he *suffered*" (Heb. 5:8).

On the eve of his final hour of suffering, Jesus gathered his disciples in an upper room and tried to prepare them for his death. But the news of his departure from this earth unsettled them. To assure them, Jesus said: "Do not let your hearts be troubled. Trust in God; trust also in me. In my Father's house are many rooms. . . . I am going there to prepare a place for you."

Life is a journey, and the one thing we all have in common is that we start out on that journey lost and disoriented. Most of us go through life distracted. Our early brushes with suffering are like a polite child who comes alongside us and tugs at our coattails to get our attention. The more suffering we experience in life, the louder and more insistent that child becomes. When we finally stop what we're doing and bend down to listen, the child whispers in our ear . . . and points the way home.

C. S. Lewis said that "the Christian doctrine of suffering explains, I believe, a very curious fact about the world we live in. The settled happiness and security which we all desire, God withholds from us by the very nature of the world: but joy, pleasure, and merriment He has scattered broadcast. We are never safe, but we have plenty of fun, and some ecstasy. It is not hard to see why. The security we crave would teach us to rest our hearts in this world and [pose] an obstacle to our return to God: a few moments of happy love, a landscape, a symphony, a merry meeting with our friends, a [swim] or a football match, have no such tendency. Our heavenly Father refreshes us on the journey with some pleasant inns, but will not encourage us to mistake them for home."

Augustine once said: "Thou hast made us for Thyself, and

our heart is restless until it rests in Thee." *Field of Dreams* is the story of a restless heart seeking rest. And so is the story of the prodigal son. Everyone's story is the story of a restless heart. We seek that rest in a lot of different inns in a lot of distant lands. But what we really long for is home.

Our Father's home.

– 29 –

I'm a Fan Now

WHEN THE GIANTS honored me at Candlestick Park with "Dave Dravecky Day," they also honored me in another way. They let me throw out the opening pitch.

For one last time in a Giants' uniform I walked onto that field in Candlestick Park. I stepped a few yards in front of the mound, wrapped my hand around the ball, felt its stitched seams with my fingers. Then, in front of 46,740 fans, this one-time finesse pitcher lobbed the ball to the catcher. And one final cheer arose for number 43.

Afterward I took my seat in the stands. It was great sitting there, but at the same time it was hard, too. Seeing all those lean athletic bodies limbering up on the field. Watching them trot off to their positions with such graceful ease. Looking at them, their hands pounding the pocket of their gloves, crouched and ready to play.

Giants' pitcher Trevor Wilson got the first two batters out. At the end of that inning, Darryl Strawberry came up to bat. Trevor threw him heat. Swing and a miss. The ballpark roared. How I used to love that roar when I was out there on that field. Two more pitches and Darryl was out. Three batters had come up to bat, and the left-hander on the mound had sent all three of them sulking toward the dugout.

"Way to go, Trevor!"

First baseman Will Clark got the first hit for the Giants. He belted a long ball into right field for a stand-up triple. Everyone in the stands jumped to their feet, cheering.

I jumped and cheered, too.

I was a fan now. And it felt good.

During the course of the day, a lot of other fans came by to talk. They thanked me for the memories, expressed their love, wished me well. A lot of them had seen my comeback game and remarked how much it meant to them.

It made me realize that when I was out there on the mound in my comeback game, I wasn't out there alone. I was out there with every other person who had faced adversity and who had the opportunity to overcome it. Now I am without my arm, without the possibility of making a comeback, and I'm not alone there, either. A lot of people are standing with me who don't have the opportunity to overcome their adversity. I hope that for those people my story has been an encouragement. I hope they realize that even though they can't overcome their adversity, they can find the grace to endure it, and they can find peace.

Many of the fans I talked with at Candlestick Park were saddened by what cancer had done to my life. They didn't say it in so many words, but you could see it in their eyes and hear it in their voices. They thought it was a tragedy.

I don't feel that way. There is a scene in *Field of Dreams* where Ray Kinsella tracked down an old ballplayer named "Moonlight" Graham. Graham's career in the major leagues was so short it wasn't even a flash in the pan. He played only a few minutes of one game in the majors, and he never got a chance to bat. That was decades ago. Graham was an old man now. He had become a doctor and had given his life to alleviate what suffering he could in the small town where he lived. They talked about his experiences as a doctor, and then the conversation turned to baseball. Kinsella couldn't get over how short Graham's career was: "For five minutes you were *that* close to your dream. It would kill some men to be that close to their dream and not to touch it; they'd consider it a tragedy."

Graham looked him in the eye and with a wistful smile said: "Son, if I'd have been a doctor for only five minutes, now that would have been a tragedy."

When I look back over the past four years and see all I've learned from other people who have suffered, all I've experienced of other people's love, all God has shown me of his mercy and comfort, all the encouragement my small measure of suffering has given to others, I think: *If I'd have continued on as a ballplayer and missed that, now that would have been a tragedy.*

THANK YOU—each and every one of you—for all your kind words, all your prayers, and the many expressions of love you have shown Jan and me in our afflictions over the past few years.

May the Father of all mercies comfort you in whatever affliction comes your way.

May he give you the strength to turn your setbacks into comebacks.

And when you can't come back, may he give you the grace to put your hand in his—even if you have only one hand to give—and there may you find peace.

Epilogue

ONE VERY IMPORTANT message has come through clearly as I have worked closely with Dave and Jan for the last few years: They sincerely want to help others. Many people have reached out to them for help since Dave's successful comeback in the summer of 1989. Many more have done so since Dave had his arm amputated in June of '91.

After reading their story, you can see why it has been difficult for them to respond to all the letters they have received since August 1989. However, the Draveckys sincerely want to answer those pleas from victims and their families for help with cancer, amputation, depression, or other crises similar to those which Dave and Jan have experienced. Therefore in addition to writing this book, they have taken specific steps to assist them in responding.

First, the Draveckys and their friends and supporters have formed THE DAVE DRAVECKY FOUNDATION, a non-profit, charitable organization that will meet the needs of those who look to Dave and Jan for some word of encouragement and hope. The Foundation office is located in the Draveckys' hometown, and they can be reached at the following address: P.O. Box 3505, Boardman, Ohio 44513.

Second, since neither Dave nor Jan receive any compensation from THE DAVE DRAVECKY FOUNDATION, Dave earns his living by accepting a few of the many speaking invitations extended to him. But there are many more invitations than can possibly be accepted. To bring their encouraging message to as many people as possible, Dave and Jan have teamed up with ProServ Television and Zondervan Publishing House to produce and distribute a feature-length documentary film of their lives. The film will help Dave and Jan share their message with many, many more than they could ever reach in person. The film is available for rental, and anyone interested can get answers to their questions by calling Zondervan at 1-800-727-8004.

Dave played in the Buick Invitational Pro Am Golf Tournament in San Diego in February 1992. Who knows, he may become a professional golfer! However, for the foreseeable future, Dave plans to spend his working hours in efforts to serve others through his speaking and ministry with the Dravecky Foundation. Jan plans to spend her working hours as a full-time wife and mother, and she will give part-time service to the Dravecky Foundation, speaking on a very occasional basis.

Sealy Yates
Orange, California

Notes

Chapter 4 – *Surgery*
[1]Albert Schweitzer, *Out of My Life & Thought*, "Epilogue" (New York: Henry Holt and Company, 1933), p. 280.

Chapter 9 – *Which Way Is Up?*
[1]Albert Schweitzer, *Reverence for Life*, "Creative Suffering" (New York: Harper & Row, Publishers, 1969), pp. 18–19.
[2]Katherine Paterson, *Gates of Excellence* (New York: Elsevier/Nelson Books, 1981), pp. 97–98.

Chapter 11 – *Calling Out to God*
[1]Hannah Hurnard, *Hinds' Feet on High Places* (Wheaton, Ill.: Tyndale House Publishers, Inc., 1975), pp. 172–73.

Chapter 20 – *"Why Does God Make You Suffer?"*
[1]C. S. Lewis, *A Grief Observed* (New York: Bantam Books, 1976), p. 5.

Chapter 21 – *The Questions That Suffering Raises*
[1]Nicholas Wolterstorff, *Lament for a Son* (Grand Rapids, Mich.: Wm. B. Eerdmans Publishing Co., 1987), pp. 67–68.
[2]C. S. Lewis, *A Grief Observed*, pp. 4–5, 53–54, 80–81.

Chapter 22 – *The Missing Pieces in Suffering*
[1]Corrie ten Boom with John and Elizabeth Sherrill, *The Hiding Place* (Old Tappan, N.J.: Fleming H. Revell Co., 1971), pp. 26–27.

Chapter 26 – *Finding the Grace*
[1]Corrie ten Boom, *The Hiding Place*, p. 29.